# Circuit Training for Weight Loss

*"Circuit Training for Beginners" +*
*"Intermediate Circuit Training" +*
*"High Intensity Circuit Training".*

*The Simple Home Workout Guide to*
*get from Fat to Fit.*

# Andrew Hudson

are declared or implied. Readers acknowledge that the author is not engaging in the rendering of legal, financial, medical or professional advice. The content within this book has been derived from various sources. Please consult a licensed professional before attempting any techniques outlined in this book.

By reading this document, the reader agrees that under no circumstances is the author responsible for any losses, direct or indirect, which are incurred as a result of the use of the information contained within this document, including, but not limited to, — errors, omissions, or inaccuracies.

# Table of Contents

# Circuit Training for Beginners

*A 6 Week Beginner Home Workout Manual for Losing Weight, Gaining Energy, and Improving Self-Esteem.*

**Andrew Hudson**

# Introduction

Many people across the world struggle with obesity or being overweight, and the problems that come with it are starting to become normal for a large chunk of the population. There are many possible reasons for why so many people are out of shape, the main ones being that unhealthy takeaways can be ordered just with a few clicks, having a healthy diet is portrayed as torture and most people don't know what it takes to lose weight.

The reasons above are just some of the reasons why 71.6% of the US population are overweight, that's almost three quarters! This means that most people in the US have thrown away their good health and now struggle with the consequence like, being more likely to develop fatal health-related issues, lack lots of energy by carrying around their excess weight and may be embarrassed by their own body.

If you feel as if you relate to any of the problems above or are worried about your health deteriorating, don't worry because this book will help you make the changes you need to escape the downsides of obesity or being overweight. I was once overweight and I know what it is like to experience some of the downsides that come with it, it was a tough time of my life and I thought breaking free from my unhealthy lifestyle was impossible. That's until I followed simple steps you can find in this book which began my weight loss journey.

I understand many people want to get out of their unhealthy lifestyle and lose weight to look better, feel more confident, or want to train for something like the army, or just lower the health risks. Whatever the reason is for you wanting to lose weight, I am here to support you along your journey.

My name is Andrew Hudson. I am a personal trainer who has recently taken a turn to writing because I know that I can help more people reach their fitness goals. I love helping people reach fitness goals for many reasons, mostly because I feel great when I see people manage to turn their life around for the good through fitness. That is also why I want to help you, although this isn't a 1 on 1 training session, you will still be able to progress towards your goal and feel great while doing so!

Circuit training is what this book is based on and it's a brilliant training method! This is because circuit training allows you can be exercise at home with little equipment, takes hardly any time to set up and is a quick workout that you can easily fit in a few times a week. Also, these circuits are quite fun if I do say so myself. This book will provide you with some great motivational tips, dietary advice, health & fitness information, weight loss tips and a wide range of exercises that will accelerate your weight loss progression.

The 6-week workout plan is what I hope for you to follow. This will gently ease you into a routine of exercise and a healthy lifestyle which will set you up for your healthy future. It doesn't end after 6 weeks because the information provided in this book will allow you to extend your routine further until you reach your fitness goal!

Exercising, learning, and breaking into a routine gets harder with age. That is why you should start now – you will not regret it! If you don't make this change now, then your health will only continue to decline, your body will not thank you for that in the future.

Your journey starts here, I wish you the best of luck and this book is your guide to your goals. Work at your own pace and follow the tips provided, I believe in you. If you are still sat on the fence, why not give this a go? You have nothing to lose...

**Circuit Training for Weight Loss**

This is the first book from the three-part series, "Circuit Training for Weight Loss". This series is for people that are looking to reach fitness goals at home with the training method: Circuit Training. Whether your goal is to lose weight to avoid health risks, to improve your health or if you are looking to lower your body fat percentage to look ripped/toned, then this series will help you out. Below you will find a brief description of each book and a summary of the series at the end, if you want to find out more, then search up the book titles to view the detailed description!

As this is the first book of this series, it is the most basic, but that doesn't mean that you won't be able to lose weight from it! This book is to get you into a simple exercise routine, will help you clean up your diet and give you an understanding of general health and fitness. This book is a great starting point to set you off on your weight loss journey, helping you break your old unhealthy habits so you can no longer fall under the obese or overweight category.

The second book of the series, "Intermediate Circuit Training", is the next step that increases the difficulty of the workouts, so you make quicker progress towards harder fitness goals. This still sticks with the theme of weight loss with circuit training and nutrition, but this book starts to branch out to slightly more advanced health & fitness information and starts to present motivational advice, so you stay on track with your fitness goal. This isn't for complete beginners, more for the average person looking to lose weight.

The final book, "High Intensity Circuit Training", is the most advanced book. The workouts in these books are shorter, but much more difficult because this book is to help people with difficult fitness goals. Goals like having a low body fat percentage and having a high lean muscle mass percentage are what can be reached by following this final book. This book also offers advice on how to adapt your mindset to reach challenging goals, information about how to boost your metabolic rate and many other ways to burn fat quickly to lower your body fat percentage while building lean muscle mass. This is for the more experienced fitness fanatics.

As you can see, each book from this series is like a steppingstone towards your final fitness goal. Each book goes up in difficulty and if you are looking to go from Fat to Fit, I highly recommend following each book 1 at a time to reach and maintain your goal of having your dream body!

# Your Free Gift

The gift you'll receive is an eBook titled: The Circuit Training Weight Loss Bundle. This eBook contains many extras to help you lose weight at a quicker rate and be on top of your progress. In the beginner section of this book, you'll discover:

2 Extra Circuits that you can complete at home, these circuits are slightly more advanced than the ones provided in this book to encourage progression.

Secondly, you will find a checklist full of the optional equipment included in this book. Each piece of equipment has a link to where you can buy it a reasonable price. A list of all the optional equipment all linked. This will allow you to find the equipment for a reasonable price.

You will also find a food budget tracker - a spreadsheet that will allow you to keep track of how much you spend on food with the goal to help you save money in a healthy fashion.

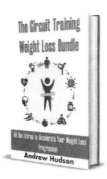

Follow this link for the free eBook:

https://hudsonandrew.activehosted.com/f/33

# Join the Workout for Weight Loss Community

Living a healthy lifestyle is difficult, especially when you feel as if you are doing it all alone. That's why I suggest for you to join a community of others who are in your situation, this community "Workout for Weight Loss" will provide you with daily posts about weight loss and there will be many people that you can talk to, share experiences with and receive help from.

I aim to post twice a day, providing you with tips, tricks, motivation, workouts, diet plans and so much more to help you lose weight. Not to mention that I may host a few book giveaways every now and then. In a community, your chance of reaching your goals is much stronger and you may make many new friends in the process!

So, if you are looking for that extra help, please join my Free Facebook Group: https://www.facebook.com/groups/workoutforweightloss

# Free "Circuit Training for Weight Loss" eBook

You may find that in this book there are a few links for you to follow which is inconvenient because you can follow a link through a paperback book without spending 10 minutes typing in 40-character links into your URL.

The links in this book are beneficial to help you progress further with your boxing ability and I don't want you to miss out on them. That is why I am giving you the free PDF eBook copy of this book so that you can access all the links with just a click.

To get the eBook, you will have to type in a short link into your URL (ironic I know…) and you will have the eBook emailed directly to your inbox.

So please type this short link into your internet browser to have easier access to links in this book:

https://hudsonandrew.activehosted.com/f/31

# Health Check

Before you start this fitness routine - please consult with your doctor.

- Do not attempt to exercise while unwell.
- Do not carry-on exercising if you feel pain - if the pain doesn't calm please tell your doctor.
- Avoid exercising after consuming alcohol or a large meal within the last couple of hours.
- If you take prescribed medication, check with your doctor to make sure it is okay to exercise.
- If you are in any doubt, go check with a doctor. It may be helpful to show the doctor the circuit training routines you will partake in, if the doctor suggests for you not to partake in certain exercises

there are always alternatives that will suit you.

Think before you train. If you are under 16 years old, then I advise you to stay away from lifting weights as your body hasn't fully developed. I 'Andrew Hudson' will not take any responsibility for any physical injuries caused by exercises I have stated in this book – injuries are a part of fitness and can always be avoided so please train responsibly.

Read through the entire book before performing any of the circuits/warmups/cooldowns.

# Chapter 1 – Why an Unhealthy Lifestyle is Miserable

Fat is not fun. Most people that are overweight want to lose weight once they realize their way of living is doing themselves some serious harm to them mentally and physically. The reason I say that not all overweight people want to lose weight is because some people are unaware of their lifestyle and some people just enjoy being a massive lump on a massive sofa. If you are reading this book, then I know you are with the majority looking to lose weight. Before you get to the "how to lose weight" part of this book, it is important you know why you need to lose weight and you can use this as motivation for any of the days that you don't feel like getting a workout in or when you're tempted for a quick chocolate bar.

This chapter will lay out why an unhealthy lifestyle is so bad for you and will give you an insight to how your lifestyle will improve once you make changes. I also urge any of you that have friends or family that are overweight but unaware of their weight, to just let them know about their unhealthy ways in a kind manner. Many people don't know that they are damaging their mind and body, just a quick heads up is all it takes is just a quick word to them which will help them out. But if you are unaware of what obesity/ being overweight does to you, you are about to find out...

## The Problem of Obesity

The term obese is described as "Grossly fat or overweight", would you be proud of being known as grossly fat?

Everyone falls under these four categories. These categories are underweight, healthy weight, overweight and obese. Your actions in life are what allow you to end up in each of these categories, actions such as eating well and exercising regularly will put you in the healthy weight class and actions like over-eating and exercising once a blue moon will most likely put you in the overweight or obese class.

BMI (Body Mass Index) is how you are measured to be placed in these groups. To calculate your BMI all you need to do is divide your weight in Kg, by your height squared in meters (Weight(kg) / Height$^2$ (m)). For this book

I want you to use your weight and BMI to track your progress, I think BMI is a great way to track progress as the number is generated from your height and weight, so it is fair to compare with other people at different weights and heights.

If your BMI is between 18.5 and 25 then congratulations, you are considered a healthy weight – a great goal for those looking to get into good shape and also a good goal for those maintaining weight. But please remember just because you are in this weight class, that doesn't mean that you're immune to becoming fat. All it takes in an unhealthy lifestyle to grow out of a healthy weight, so once you reach this BMI, remember to maintain it.

Underweight BMI – If your BMI is below 18.5 then you are underweight. You will want to gain weight, both muscle mass and body fat. If you find yourself in this situation, this book won't help you. Instead, increase your portion sizes and start body weight training.

Overweight BMI – If you have a BMI that is between 25 and 30, unfortunately, you are considered overweight and will need to cut the fat. Luckily, you are currently reading a book that will allow you to cut the pounds so that you get back into the healthy weight section.

Obese BMI – A BMI above 30 means you are obese. Hopefully, if you are in this zone then you will study this book to make a change. There is always time to slim up and lower your BMI, carry on reading and get stuck in!

It's finally time to get into the problems that come with being overweight or obese. These problems are mostly health-related issues, and I cannot say that you are guaranteed to fall victim to them because of your weight, but I can say that the higher your BMI is above 25 then the more likely you will be at a high risk to these fatal health conditions. The health-related problems include:

- Increased chance of cancer.
- High Blood Pressure.
- Increased risk of stroke.
- Increased risk of heart disease.
- Higher chance of Kidney Disease.

I listed the most common and fatal ones but believe me when I say the list doesn't end there. I hope that makes you aware of the danger you are in from your current situation. This should be scary and proves that the benefits of being overweight, which is just being able to be a couch potato, are heavily outweighed by the negatives. If the previous conditions weren't a big enough wake-up call, then I will list a few more mental problems caused by being overweight.

- More likely to be stressed
- Low self-esteem
- Low confidence in certain situations

Yet again just the most common problems listed but that should be enough for you to reconsider your food choices and your lifestyle. If that's not enough to persuade you, there is more to hopefully make you see that your current unhealthy lifestyle isn't working out for you.

The 71.6% of American that are overweight are more likely to need hospital treatment because of their lifestyle, which of course isn't ideal or cheap. This is likely to put you under financial stress, which can be easily avoided from a change to your lifestyle.

Finally, I would like to say how a healthy diet is much cheaper than having all these takeaways and snacks. Although I am going to contradict myself by saying that studies have proved healthy food to be more expensive than unhealthy food. However, it is typical for unhealthy food to be less filling and more addictive which causes the consumer to buy more unhealthy foods. If you look at the prices of takeaways, you can see how quickly they add up to put a dent in your bank balance. A healthy diet contains more filling food which will keep your energy levels high, won't require you to buy too much and will save you money. Later on in this book, the diet section proves how that is the case with examples.

**Benefits of Living Healthy**

Let me guess, you think that being healthy is awful because of all the general stereotypes that suggest healthy people wake up with a glass of that disgusting green juice and go on a run every day. Well, I want to use this book to prove that's not the case, you can still enjoy the grub every now and then but once you are in the routine of living healthy you will appreciate the switch you made. Here are just some benefits of being healthy that should encourage you to make the switch:

- Feeling more confident.
- Looking slimmer.
- Having more energy.
- Reduces the chance of dementia.
- Reduces the chance of osteoporosis.
- Gives you clear skin.

Doesn't that sound so much better! By exercising and eating well you are expanding your life expectancy and improving the quality of your life. This all doesn't come instantly, you have to give it time and stick to it but I promise you that the results will come.

## My Experience of Health & Fitness

I will just give you a brief history of myself, how I was affected by being overweight and how exercise changed my life.

Many years ago, I was fat. My BMI was 26.3 and I always found myself drained of energy after work. Working long days would leave me no choice but to eat junk and train only on the weekends with low energy. I failed countless times at exercising and I would give up midsession, that was because I had insufficient energy levels and couldn't motivate myself to stick to it.

As a simple man, I hated seeing all these weight loss videos on fasting or certain diets, I just wanted a routine I could follow to get myself out of my poor situation. I remember circuit training sessions from school and made many circuits with exercises that I know would make me sweat. After following these workouts and started cutting the junk out of my diet, I got into boxing and found my love for fitness.

As the years have gone by, I no longer struggle with low-confidence levels, being ashamed of my body and being unable to motivate myself. It was thrilling to see how the years of exercise had bettered me as a person, which is why I want to better everyone who reads my books. As a qualified personal trainer and a boxing coach, I enjoy teaching others and I only hope to reach more and more of you out there!

# Chapter 2 – What Makes Circuit Training Great for Losing Weight

### Introduction to Circuit Training

Circuit training is a workout technique that involves a series of exercises performed in a cycle, with minimal rest in between each exercise. Circuits usually have 4 to 12 exercises in one rotation and can be repeated however many times necessary. Circuit training can be done at home, outside or at a gym. Ideally, you will need a bit of open space. Getting started is always the hardest part and I understand it takes a lot of work to do something that you think you will hate.

### Benefits of Circuit Training

Circuit training is honestly fantastic! The pros outweigh the cons by a country mile, I will list a few reasons below that support my statement:

**Circuit Training is Practical** – Set up circuit training at home, at the gym or outside without worrying. Depending on the equipment required for the circuit it is unlikely to take longer than 3 minutes to get ready and usually takes under 30 minutes to complete. This allows you to fit a training session into your busy schedule.

**Circuit Training brings Variety** – Circuit training can be set up in any way to train anything. In this book the focus is on weight loss, even though that slightly narrows down what can be trained there are still many exercises that can be used with circuit training. These exercises can be done inside and out, with or without equipment and altered to be time efficient. Here are some ways circuit training can be used for training:

- Improving Aerobic Endurance (Improving Fitness Levels)
- Building Muscular Strength (Gaining Muscle Mass)
- Improving Muscular Endurance (Improving how long muscles can take exercise before getting tired)
- Weight Loss (Burning fat at a steady rate)
- Getting back into a sport after an injury (Recovery)
- Improving anaerobic endurance (HIIT Training, intense fat burning or muscle building)

**Circuit Training is for Everyone** – That's right, whether the only exercise you do is going to the shop or whether you work out twice a day – circuit training has so many variables that you can change to make it suit you! I would suggest you stop reading this book if you work out twice a day as you will need more of a challenge, my other books may help you!

**Circuit Training is Easily Modified** – There are many changeable variables that determine how hard you train, how often you train, what you train and so on. Changing the variables is a key part of implementing Progressive Overload. I have listed the variables below:

**Circuit Training Variables:**
- Number of exercises in the circuit.
- The number of sets.
- The time spent doing each exercise.
- Reps completed for each exercise.
- The time spent resting between each station.
- How long to rest after a set.
- The resistance of the exercises.

- The intensity level you work at during the exercise station.
- What exercises to include.
- How many days a week you train.

**Circuit Training is Time-Efficient** – Circuits usually last between 20 minutes to an hour, in this book I am to make circuits last roughly 30 minutes as I understand you will struggle with long periods of exercise.

**Circuit Training allows you to stay Motivated** – There are a few ways to stay motivated using circuit training, other training methods have more limits so that some of these motivation factors wouldn't work. I will now talk about ways to stay motivated.

## Motivation

If you are reading this book the chances are that you are overweight, obese or not happy with your shape or size. The first step for change is you reading this book to learn how you can lose weight, the following steps are you exercising regularly, following a diet, staying in routine and this is all possible by staying motivated.

Being motivated is where you have a drive or passion to reach your goal every single day, even on the days or sessions where you've had enough you still push yourself to get it done. Staying motivated is hard, especially if you train by yourself – this is why I am here to offer you tips on how to feel motivated every day until you reach your goals.

Signs of becoming demotivated can be as little as not finishing the last minute of a workout.

Once you start to cut things out of your routine, you will lose weight at a slower rate or start to gain weight if you drop the routine. What I am trying to say is that you must stick to your training and diet plan for a prolonged period, so that you can see the results you are after. Of course, you will not see results after a few days of training, don't let this put you off.

**How to Stay Motivated**

Motivation is key to continue exercising on a regular basis, it can be hard to force yourself to exercise sometimes but to reach your goals or solve your problems. You have to have the correct mindset in order to continue, without it you will be lost. If you ever feel like not exercising refer to the points below and find that drive deep within yourself.

I believe that getting into a routine is the best way to motivate yourself. Have you heard the phrase '3 weeks makes a habit'? Well once you get into a habit of training you will be in a routine and get used to exercising. It may start off with just 2 days a week which is great as you are building a routine so you can work towards your fitness goals. This is my biggest goal as an author, if I can see people get into a routine then I know a strong foundation is set.

Working out with other people is also a great way to motivate yourself. You won't even realize it but when you work out with a friend or family member you will enjoy it more – a social aspect of fitness is very good as you will be excited to work out again with somebody. You could also have a friendly competition to push each other.

Reward yourself. If you reach your goal treat yourself to something like a night out with friends or family, this may push you to meet your goal. Try not to reward yourself with something that will reverse your progress like a large chocolate cake. Just have fun once your goal is reached.

Make it fun. Many people dread exercising, but if you can find a way to put your own spin on it to make it fun then please go for it as you will enjoy exercising. If you enjoy exercising, then you will have no problem with exercising making you motivated. I have tried to make the circuits involved in this book fun because why would anyone want to do something, they don't find enjoyable.

**Example Circuit**

Now that the complete basics are covered, here is how I lay out all the circuits involved in this book. I start with listing a few instructions, the first one will be how many sets to complete – this is the number of times you should complete the circuit. Secondly, I state how long to rest in between each exercise, for most circuits it is 30 seconds – please note that this not the same as the rest period between sets.

The rest between sets is longer because you need to recover to get into another circuit, I may also word this as rest for 3 minutes after completing the first set. I then set you a target of what heart rate/training zone you should work at – the previous sub-chapter explains this. I finally state the time it takes to complete the warmup, circuit and cooldown, which all play a part reaching the recommended 150 minutes of moderate physical activity.

Complete 2 sets, rest for 30 seconds between each exercise with a 3-minute rest between each set. Train at the Light Training Zone (Around 60% of Max HR). This circuit takes roughly 20 minutes to complete including the warmup and cooldown.

Warmup 1

1. Pushups – 30 seconds
2. Marching on the spot – 30 seconds
3. Calf Raise – 30 seconds
4. Half Squats – 30 seconds
5. Knees to Chest – 30 seconds
6. Jog on the spot – 30 seconds

Cooldown 1

At the top and bottom of the circuit, I include the phrase "Warmup 1" and "Cooldown 1", to avoid confusion I have that there because it should remind the reader to warm up before the circuit and cooldown after the circuit. "Warmup 1" is the name of a warmup I have provided in this book, you will need to be familiar with the warmups and cool down I provide in this book as you will be doing them before and after every circuit.

**Example Six-Week Plan**

This is just a short sub-chapter that demonstrates how I lay out my actual Six-week plan in the 7th chapter. Every day is covered, and this should be an inspiration for those who want to create their own six-week plan.

**Week 1:**

**Monday** –

What to Train: Train Example Circuit 1

Progressive Overload Changes: No changes to this circuit.

**Tuesday** – Rest Day

**Wednesday** –

What to Train: Complete Example Circuit 2

Progressive Overload Changes: No changes to this circuit.

**Thursday** – Rest Day

**Friday** –

What to Train: Train Example Circuit 1

Progressive Overload: Instead of resting for 30 seconds, march on the spot. This will keep you working for longer. Please still use the time to rest properly between the sets.

**Saturday** –

What to Train: Complete Example Circuit 2

Progressive Overload: Make a slight change to this particular circuit by working for 40 seconds on each exercise, this will make you work for longer to complete the circuit and more calories burnt.

**Sunday** – Rest Day

Week 1 Overview:

On Monday and Wednesday, you will be training the example circuits as normal. On Friday you will modify the circuit so that you spend less time resting by replacing the 30 second rest period by marching on the spot – this light activity still builds up the workload. On Saturday I use progressive overload to the second example circuit by increasing the time spent on exercises to make it harder. You have completed 120 minutes of exercise this week which is getting you closer to the recommended 150 minutes.

After the week's plan, I also include an overview of the week to reinforce the information. I do not provide a certain time for when you train, but I strongly suggest you train between two meals, so you have sufficient energy for before and after the circuit – obviously leave enough time as isn't good to train straight after eating. This is just an example so please don't follow this.

## Equipment

Don't worry, this book requires no equipment for completing the circuits. That means you won't have to spend lots of money which is always a bonus. I will list a few things that you may find helpful for when you are working out. You can find links to all the equipment for a reasonable price in the Basic Circuit Training Bundle. Please remember everything below is optional, I want to make exercising cheap as possible so that it gives more people motivation to do so.

- A Smart Watch that tracks your Heart Rate.
- A Stopwatch to help you keep track of how long you exercise for. Can use an app on your phones if it cheaper for you.
- 2kg Hand Weights that you can hold while completing the circuits to make it slightly harder.
- Fitness Matt – Just to make it more comfortable to train on the floor and stops sweat getting on the floor.

- Fitness Attire – Just a pair of shorts and a training top/bra will be suitable for when you are exercising. I link some reasonably priced brands in the basic circuit training bundle.

# Chapter 3 – You Are What You Eat

I feel as if this is the part most people are least looking forward to when it comes to making a change to live a healthy lifestyle. But it's not as bad as you may think, you will still be able to taste great food and you will feel an increase in your energy levels. Diet may be hard to stick to, but it really is important and you will learn why. After reading this, you will be aware of what a healthy diet consists of and how it is much different to what you would expect!

## The Importance of Diet

If you eat like crap, then you will train like crap – it is as simple as that. Many people underestimate the importance of how you choose to eat and drink. Training will help you get into shape, but if you are going to eat poorly then you may as well not train. A good diet goes hand in hand with training hard.

It can be easy to put on a bit of weight, I do have some sympathy for the larger people as I was once on the heavy side – working full time got me to make poor food choices. I will explain the most common ways of getting to an overweight stage below. The points below also prove a point that you are not overweight because you are unlucky, your choices in life have gotten you to where you are.

Eating poorly – Although this sounds obvious many people don't realize when they are eating poorly. For example, a sugary snack every couple of hours doesn't sound harmful – I can assure you it all adds up to be stored as fat in your body. As you can guess, the more fat stored in your body the rounder you look.

Quick Meals and Snacks – This is a big reason for the millions of overweight people. I used to work a long shift and I know that it is much easier to get microwavable meals and snacks than to prepare nutritional meals. The takeaways and snacks will not provide your body with all the nutrients that are needed, the food is mostly heavily processed, in which you know that is not good for your body.

How much you eat – Even if you eat foods that are considered healthy, it is still possible to get fat by eating too much of those foods. That is why you need to space out when you eat. It will be unrealistic to drastically cut down on how much you eat each day, that why you should eat smaller meals more often every day.

Late-night snacks – Many people think that it is bad to eat anything at night but there is nothing wrong with it. Typically, people make poor food choices later on in the day. You need to remember that calories DO count at night and swap the midnight brownie for a midnight banana.

Lack of exercise – Although this hasn't got much to do with diet, how you eat does affect how you train. A good diet will provide your body with energy so you can train hard. Exercising after eating foods high in saturated fat and sugar will make training very difficult and potentially make you sick – putting you off exercise.

## What Your Body Needs

Your daily diet will need to consist of:

- 30% Protein. You can get this from many things like eggs, lean meats, poultry, beans cheese and natural peanut butter.

- 30% Fats. Good fats that contain omega-3 and omega-6 fatty acids are essential for bone, joint, and brain health. Good sources of these fatty acids include fish, nuts, olive oil, flax seeds, or avocados.

- 40% Carbohydrates. Natural carbs like peas, sweet potatoes, beans, nuts, and whole grains.

- 25 grams of Fiber. Fiber helps with digestion and regulating weight. Foods high in fiber are things like fruits, vegetables, whole oats, nuts, and legumes. Many people struggle to consume this much. Fiber is wonderful because it keeps you full up for longer.

- 2.5 liters of water. It is important to stay hydrated, after all, your body is made up of 70% water

Everything that I mentioned above fuels the body's metabolism. It is important that you understand how the metabolism works, in the subchapter underneath I compare the human body to a furnace as it will help you understand the importance of your diet.

## How the Metabolism Works

*The Furnace Analogy:*

The body is just like a fire, it needs fuel to get started. With a fire you need paper, firelighters, sticks, logs and coal to keep it burning. You light the paper to set fire to the firelighters to set fire to the sticks and so on to get to the coal. This will keep the fire lit in the furnace to keep you warm all day. Now let's substitute some things to compare this furnace to your body. Instead of paper you have vitamins, instead of the firelighters you have minerals, instead of sticks we have protein, instead of logs we have carbs and finally instead of coal we have fats. The body needs vitamins, minerals, proteins, carbs and fats to keep the metabolism working hard so that you have enough energy for your body to function to the best of its ability all day long.

**The Most Important Meal of the Day**

Did your mum tell you that breakfast is the most important meal of the day? Well, your mum is always right after all. A survey showed a couple of years back that 98% of people that live in the UK said they either don't eat breakfast, or they eat what is considered an unhealthy breakfast. Although the percentage may have changed slightly as it's now 2021, this still isn't good enough and links heavily to people generally having no energy all day long.

A healthy balanced breakfast is so important in the morning, think of a healthy breakfast like lighting the fire. The correct breakfast choice will kickstart your day with all the nutrients you need to energize your body – this will allow you to not find yourself tired after waking up and feeling great throughout the day.

Overall, you should take from this that you need to have a healthy breakfast every day and you need to space out meals to keep your energy levels high. If you have low energy all day long you will struggle at work, or to exercise and make things harder for yourself.

## Weight Loss Tips

The overall idea of a weight loss diet is to eat a balanced diet and to eat less than your daily recommended calorie intake – for Men: 2500 calories, for Women: 2000 calories. Here are a few tips to consider that will help with weight loss:

- Eat lots of Leafy Green vegetables like kale, spinach, and collards are low in calories and contain a lot of fiber.
- Stay away from eating junk food, allow yourself a cheat day once a fortnight.
- Structure out what you will eat every day, leave 3 hours between each time you eat.
- Try to eat less for each meal but make up for it by having 5 meals a day, 3 of them should be the main meals and 2 of them should be mini meals in between the mains.
- Avoid snacking regularly, snack once or twice a day. Snack on healthy foods like nuts, or protein shakes. Don't tempt yourself with a chocolate bar.

What you should gather from this section is to cut out junk food from your diet, you should ideally have 5 meals a day and have 2 snacks at the most. Fill up your dinner plate with leafy vegetables. Most importantly you should track what you eat every day, track calories by using the app MyFitnessPal on your phone or you can find a calorie tracker spreadsheet in the Basic Circuit Training Bundle.

**Eating Before and After Training**

Eating before and after training is very important as you will have to fuel your body to perform the exercises and it is recommended to replenish your body with energy and nutrients after a workout. Eat a small nutritional meal roughly an hour before a workout and eat a bigger meal after a workout. A small meal could be like natural Greek yogurt with berries and a larger meal could be like half a chicken breast with pasta in sauce. If you are struggling for motivation, then check out the weeks diet plan.

**Diet Plan**

For this section, I will include a week's diet plan that you can follow throughout the six-weeks. This is likely to be a big change from your normal diet, instead of me slowly cutting down your snacks and diet I want you to get straight into it and build a healthy habit. Feel free to replace any meals with what suits you – as long as it isn't any junk. This diet plan is suitable for men and women that are planning to lose weight.

Firstly, I would like to start by saying that for every day, you need to consume 2.5 liters of water. This is very important for keeping you hydrated. Secondly, you will need to figure out what your recommended daily calorie intake is. You are all different shapes and sizes which means you need to consume a different number of calories every day to keep your body energized. Please follow this link to discover what your recommended calorie intake is.

https://www.calculator.net/calorie-calculator.html

All you have to do is type in your height and weight, then 4 numbers will pop up, these are recommended calorie intakes. As you are looking to lose weight, I strongly suggest you aim to consume either one of the bottom two figures – either weight loss or extreme weight loss. Now you know how many calories you are aiming to consume every day to lose weight.

This diet plan unfortunately will not be specific to you, unless you happen to require the same number of daily calories as the diet plan provides. I have tried my best to make this a one size fits all diet plan, if the daily calories for this plan exceeds or falls short of your daily recommended calorie intake, please make changes where necessary by increasing or decreasing portion sizes. Please don't feel forced into following this exact plan if you have any allergies or intolerances, there are many alternative healthy meals out there so feel free to make any replacements. This diet plan is just something for you to take inspiration from.

Diet plan: Split up into 5 meals a day with room for one or two snacks. Each day of eating contains roughly 1800 calories. Two cheat meals allowed all week, they are both on Sunday. I also suggest for you to take vitamin and mineral tablets every day. After a while you will get close to reaching your fitness goal, when you get close to the weight you want to achieve you should start to increase your calorie intake slightly, so you don't continue losing weight until you look like a twig.

**Monday –**

Breakfast (6am-9am): Bowl of Oatmeal with Your Choice of Toppings

Mid-Morning Meal (9am-12pm): Two slices of whole meal buttered toast with a choice of fruit.

Lunch (12pm-3pm): Healthy Lunch Meal

Midafternoon Meal (3pm-6pm): Baked Beans on Toast – Use 2 slices of whole meal bread.

Dinner (6pm-9pm): Healthy Evening Meal

Snacks (Any time): 2 Snacks – Protein Bar & 30 grams of mixed nuts.

**Tuesday –**

Breakfast (6am-9am): Bowl of Oatmeal with Your Choice of Toppings

Mid-Morning Meal (9am-12pm): Two slices of whole meal buttered toast with a choice of fruit.

Lunch (12pm-3pm): Healthy Lunch Meal

Midafternoon Meal (3pm-6pm): Coriander, Chicken and Rice.

Dinner (6pm-9pm): Healthy Evening Meal

Snacks (Any time): 1 Snack - Protein Shake

**Wednesday –**

Breakfast (6am-9am): Bowl of Oatmeal with Your Choice of Toppings

Mid-Morning Meal (9am-12pm): Two slices of whole meal buttered toast with a choice of fruit.

Lunch (12pm-3pm): Healthy Lunch Meal.

Midafternoon Meal (3pm-6pm): Chicken Soup.

Dinner (6pm-9pm): Healthy Evening Meal.

Snacks (Any time): 2 Snacks – Protein Bar & Greek yogurt with mixed berries.

**Thursday –**

Breakfast (6am-9am): Bowl of Oatmeal with Your Choice of Toppings

Mid-Morning Meal (9am-12pm): Two slices of whole meal buttered toast with a choice of fruit.

Lunch (12pm-3pm): Healthy Lunch Meal

Midafternoon Meal (3pm-6pm): Cajan Rice Bake

Dinner (6pm-9pm): Healthy Evening Meal

Snacks (Any time): 1 Snack – Just the Protein Shake.

**Friday –**

Breakfast (6am-9am): Bowl of Oatmeal with Your Choice of Toppings

Mid-Morning Meal (9am-12pm): Two slices of whole meal buttered toast with a choice of fruit.

Lunch (12pm-3pm): Healthy Lunch Meal

Midafternoon Meal (3pm-6pm): Instant Pot Chicken and Rice

Dinner (6pm-9pm): Healthy Evening Meal

Snacks (Any time): 2 Snacks – 30 grams of mixed nuts x2

**Saturday –**

Breakfast (6am-9am): Bowl of Oatmeal with Your Choice of Toppings

Mid-Morning Meal (10am-11.30am): Two slices of whole meal buttered toast with a choice of fruit.

Lunch (12pm-2pm): Healthy Lunch Meal

Midafternoon Meal (2.30pm-4:30pm): Chicken and Rice with Broccoli Pesto

Dinner (5.30pm-8:30pm): Healthy Evening Meal

Snacks (Any time): 2 Snacks – Apple Slices with Peanut Butter & 30 grams of Mixed Nuts.

**Sunday –**

Breakfast (6am-9am): Bowl of Oatmeal with Your Choice of Toppings

Mid-Morning Meal (9am-12pm): Two slices of whole meal buttered toast with a choice of fruit.

Lunch (12pm-3pm): Cheat Meal

Midafternoon Meal (3pm-6pm): Half a chicken breast, chopped and seasoned with 100 grams of basmati rice.

Dinner (6pm-9pm): Cheat Meal.

Snacks (Any time): 1 Snack – Protein Bar.

**Diet Plan Overview:**

The breakfast is the same every day, but oatmeal gives you that slow releasing energy you need to start your day properly. This will provide you with 200-300 calories, depending on your topping and what milk you mix the oats with. If oatmeal is not your go to meal, you will find a couple of alternatives later on, but most healthy breakfasts have a combination of oats, fruit and a dairy product.

The Mid-Morning Meal is the same meal every day. Two bits of toast buttered with a side of fruit. This is just an energy boost to fill you up until lunch. This meal is around 200-300 calories depending on the fruit – I personally suggest a banana. Treat this meal as a heavy snack, yet again sorry for the lack of variety for your mornings but you can always search up healthy brunch ideas if you are ever feeling bored. This meal would contain 200-300 calories.

Lunch is the meal for the middle of your day, should provide you with plenty of energy and protein. The lunch meals below should fall around 300-400 calories per serving. You can find many examples of what make a healthy lunch meal under the title "Healthy Lunch Meals", so keep reading to find them and fill up your diet plan!

The Mid-afternoon meal is just another light meal to keep you going until dinner, this usually contains a light chicken dish with a side of rice/veg/pasta but remember you can make adjustments if you don't like what is described on the diet plan. This meal offers roughly 200-400 calories and will keep your energy levels high.

Dinner is the final meal of the day and should be the biggest. As you can probably see by looking at the diet plan, it just states Healthy Evening Meal. You will find a large variety of evening meals that can fill in that spot in the diet plan, pick out some of the meals that you think look good. This meal should contain roughly 400 calories with a high amount of protein.

Snacks are also optional; I would certainly have no more than 2 a day and keep them healthy. You can find snacking options later on in this chapter for inspiration, the snacks will range from 200 to 400 calories. Snack whenever you feel like you need an energy boost, I would suggest that you snack after dinner or snack around your workout if you are exercising that day – I will state more information on when to train in the six-week plan for each day. I also suggest splitting up your snacks – by this I mean that you don't have both snacks in one sitting.

**Healthy Meal Alternatives**

Most days in the Diet plan repeat "Healthy Lunch Meal" and "Healthy Evening Meal". This doesn't really mean anything when reading it the first time, but you will find all the meals that fit under this category. The reason I structured this chapter like this is so that you have plenty of alternatives for each meal without getting confused. If you are reading from the Print Copy, I suggest for you to download the free eBook that comes with this so you can easily access all the links. Alternatively, you can go to the references to type in the link or search each individual meal listed.

**Breakfast alternatives:**

Granola with yogurt and berries

Healthy cereal that includes Muesli, Bran flakes, cornflakes. (Roughly 190 calories per serving with milk)

**Healthy Lunch Meals:**

Tomato Quinoa Soup

Charred Shrimp and Avocado Salad

Grilled Steak Tortilla Salad

Tapas Salad

Butternut Squash and White Bean Soup

Grilled Chicken Sliders

Summer Minestrone

Roasted Salmon with Green Beans and Tomatoes

Crispy Tofu Bowl

Summer Pesto Pasta

Very basic quick meals (What I tend to eat almost every day):

Chicken and rice – Half a chicken breast chopped and seasoned with 100g of basmati rice.

Sausage and Pasta in tomato sauce – Two sausages with around 100g of pasta in a tomato sauce that I get from the shop. Very basic but also tasty.

**The recipes for the meals I have included are below:**

Baked Beans on Toast – Very simple. Heat beans in a saucepan, toast whole meal bread then butter the toast and put it all together.

Coriander Chicken and Rice

Instant Pot Chicken and Rice

Cajan Rice Bake

Chicken Soup – I think the tins of chicken soup from the supermarkets are easy and affordable to prepare and eat.

Chicken and Rice with Broccoli Pesto

Half a chicken breast chopped and seasoned with 100 grams of basmati rice – This is my personal favorite, I use "chicken seasoning" that can be found in supermarkets and it takes 10 mins to prepare.

I want to include the most options for dinner as eating the same thing each week can get boring. In the plan I list "Healthy Evening Meal" – this is very broad and doesn't exactly tell you what to eat. That's why I am going to list many meals below that fall under that category, you can simply just prepare and eat the meals that I list below. I will also link a recipe with the meal, I am not exactly a cook myself so I will not list difficult recipes. Calories for dinner range between 200-500 calories. (The recipes are from UK websites so keep that in mind for the measurements)

**Healthy Evening Meals:**

Vegetable Burritos

Healthy Chicken Casserole (390 Calories)

Courgette Pasta Bake

Weight Watcher Cajun chicken recipe

Chili con Carne

Spring Chicken Soup

Ground Turkey Bolognese

Cheesesteak stuffed peppers

Skinny Alfredo

Honey Walnut Shrimp

Thai Style Chicken Salad

Cauliflower Mac n' Cheese

Crispy Chicken with Roasted Carrots and Couscous

California Chicken Flatbread with Chipotle Ranch

Honey Garlic Salmon

Cheat Meal – Can be anything you please because you deserve it. I allow two cheat meals a week, I believe that is fair and won't reverse your weight loss progress. Calories unknown – that's for you to record. Although this is a cheat meal, don't go over the top by eating triple what you would usually eat in a day because you would most likely throw that back up!

Keep in mind the serving sizes of the recipes above. You can substitute other ingredients if you feel like it works. I thought I would provide these links to offer you variety, but you can be like me and live off chicken, rice and vegetables. I like to add leafy green vegetables to all my meals, so maybe you can as well. Now you have so many options which should end your takeaway habits.

**Healthy Snacking Options:**
- Protein Bar (140 calories)
- Protein Drink Mix (108 calories)
- 30g Mixed Nuts (Around 200 calories)

- Apple Slices with peanut butter (200 calories) – 1 medium apple with 15g of natural peanut butter.
- Greek Yogurt with Mixed Berries (150 calories) – 100g of natural Greek yogurt and 50g of berries.

# Chapter 4 – What to do Before and After Exercise

Before you get into the circuits, you must know how you can prepare for them. It is not advisable to get straight into a circuit, going straight into an workout (circuit) is risky because you are more prone to injury. It is just as important to look after yourself after a workout by completing a cooldown. I will list 2 easy warmups and 1 cooldown that you can use before and after each circuit.

**Warmups**

Before each workout, it is important that you complete a warmup. The idea of a warmup is to loosen up the muscles and slowly raise your heart rate to get you ready for exercise. A typical warmup should include heart raisers and stretches which usually lasts 3 to 5 minutes. I will list a couple of different warmups below that you can complete before a weight loss circuit. I have included how to complete all the warmup exercises in Chapter 8.

Warmup 1 (3 Minutes) – Should be very light.
- Walking on the spot – 30 seconds
- Arm Swings – 30 seconds
- Overhead Triceps Stretch – 15 seconds each arm
- Child's Pose – 30 seconds
- Standing Hamstring Stretch – 15 seconds each leg

This warmup will need to be completed before the Very Low Impact Circuits 1 and 2.

Warmup 2 (4 Minutes) – Should be a light warmup.
- Marching on Spot – 1 minute

- Arm Circles – 30 seconds
- Left Right Floor Taps - 1 minute
- Quad Stretch – 15 seconds each leg
- Cross Body Shoulder Stretch – 15 seconds each arm
- Chest Expansion – 30 seconds

You should be completing this warmup before the Low Impact circuits and the Medium Impact Circuit.

## Cooldowns

Cooldowns take place after the workout and typically last 3-5 minutes. Cooldowns allow gradual recovery of heart rate and blood pressure. Cooldowns help you relax after a workout so that your recovery time will improve. Cooldown exercises range from light activity to seated stretches. I will list a simple cooldown below. Remember to check chapter 8 for the exercise descriptions. This should be completed after every circuit.

Cooldown 1 (3 Minutes) – Aim to lower your heart rate slowly.

- Light March on Spot – 30 seconds
- Close the Gates – 30 seconds
- Shoulder Shrugs – 30 seconds
- Shake off the body – 30 seconds
- Seated Spinal Twists – 30 seconds
- Seated Hamstring Stretch – 15 seconds each leg

**Rest and Recovery**

Tips to help with recovery:

- Replenish Fluids. During a workout, your body will use up lots of fluid for energy. You ideally need to refill during exercise but if you replenish after you will get a great recovery boost. Replenishing fluids is like drinking water or healthy supplements such as protein shakes.

- Resting and relaxing - You need to allow your body time to recover after a workout, this is because your muscles are likely to be slightly damaged after a workout – if you continue to train on the slightly damaged muscle then you will make the damage worse and put yourself at risk of an injury. Hopefully, you know how to rest and relax – may just be like sitting around at home.

- Cooldown – Just covered this but a good cooldown will lower the chance of injury and keep the muscles in good condition.

- Ice bath – May sound unpleasant but the coldness will make the muscles feel less sore.

- Water therapy – This is where you have a shower with hot water for 2 minutes and cold water for 30 seconds, repeat 4 times. The reason for that is that the difference in temperate will repeatedly constrict and dilate blood vessels to flush out waste products in the tissues.

- Sleep – Aim for 8 hours every night, your body produces growth hormones while you sleep which is mainly responsible for growth and repair.

- Avoid Overtraining – You want to train hard but not too hard, it will take your muscles longer to recover if they are extremely worn. You will also risk injury which may take you weeks to recover from.

If you are injured, then recovery is very important. Use the tips above to speed up your recovery time so you can get back into training quicker. Younger people and athletes are more likely to have a better recovery time, anyone can still improve their recovery time by training more often and using the tips. Do not try to exercise too soon after an injury or a workout as you will not have recovered and will be likely just to get an injury, be patient and slowly get back into it until you feel confident you are ready to train hard again.

As you exercise throughout your life your recovery time will progressively get better. I will suggest a few supplements that will help you with quicker recovery but it isn't exactly needed at your level. Protein is the nutrient that helps rebuild muscle so fill up on protein shakes and meat!

## Summary

Overall, exercising is more than just working out a few times a week. You will have to change the way you live essential by eating healthier and preparing for workouts by warming up and cooling down. I guarantee if you follow this you will reduce the risk of getting injured, this is a big positive as you will be able to continue circuit training and feel great about yourself for doing so.

# Chapter 5 – The Training Basics You Need to Know

This chapter will focus on helping you make progress towards your fitness goals. In this chapter, you will discover how the intensity of your workouts can be calculated, how the intensity will help you make progress, how training zones work, why progressive overload is the driving factor to making progress with weight loss and finally how to avoid injury.

## Intensity

Intensity is simply a variable in circuit training that is a measurement of how hard you are working. Intensity is a variable that can be measured by heart rate. The harder you work while exercising the higher your heart rate will be. It is known that the fitter the individual is the harder it is for them to raise their heart rate, that's why if you are overweight it will be relatively easy for you to raise your heart rate.

The ways you can work harder by exercising depends on how you are exercising. If you are running then run faster, if you are weightlifting then lift heavier and so on. For circuit training, the best way to work harder is to decrease the time spent resting between exercising and you can also try to fit in more reps in the 30 seconds of exercise or you could add an extra exercise to your circuit. There are so many ways to make it harder and that's why I love circuit training.

**Training Zones**

There are 5 training zones, each training zone determines how hard you are working while exercising. This uses your active heart rate to put you in a zone. Before training, athletes will set a goal of what training zone they will want to stay in during their workout,

**Very Light** – 50-60% of max heart rate. This is for when you slowly raise your heart rate during a warmup or for people recovering from injury. Walking is an exercise in this range.

**Light** – 60-70% of max heart rate. This is also known as the fat-burning zone. You should be able to exercise at this level for long time, this zone will help you burn fat and improve muscular endurance. A good warmup would take place in this zone.

**Moderate** – 70-80% of max heart rate. This zone is great form improving blood circulation around your heart and skeletal muscles, you will get a bit of a sweat on from this zone. Training in this zone is also good for burning fat.

**Hard** – 80-90% of max heart rate. You will breathe harder and work aerobically. At this intensity, you will improve your speed endurance and get used to having lactic acid in your blood. I do not recommend working in his zone for a long period as this may result in injury.

**Maximum** – 90-100% of max heart rate. Your body will be working at maximum capacity, you can only train in this zone for short periods of time as lactic acid builds up quickly in the blood and can cause cramp or injury. Working in this zone is unsustainable.

For this book, I suggest that you never work harder than the moderate zone (Over 80% of max HR). Start by working in the light zone and remember to use warmups to slowly raise your heart rate to the correct zone. When you look at the circuits it will state which training zone to exercise at.

## How to Calculate Heart Rate

You will need to be able to track your heart rate during exercise for you to stay on track in the same training zone. The best way to measure your heart rate is to buy a smartwatch that can measure your heart rate, it may be slightly pricey but once you have it, life will be easy as you can track your heart rate while exercising- the smartwatch may also include many other benefits that will help you with your fat burning journey. You don't have to pay for a smartwatch, you can measure by counting your pulse in a minute after the workout, but this is long and tedious.

You may be wondering why you should only work in a particular training zone, well this is because working outside of your training zone will make it too hard or too easy for you. If you find the training is too easy then you will not make any gain towards your goal of losing weight, because you will not be using as much energy your body will store that unused energy as glycogen and if too much glycogen is stored then it is stored as fat for the long term. If you end up storing more fat then you obviously won't be losing much weight. Training should be hard but not so hard that it is unbearable, if you find yourself almost breathless, on the verge of vomiting or a certain body part hurts then stop as you will just cause your body harm. This links to injury which I cover further on.

In order to work in the training zone that suits you then you will need to know your max heart rate. You can work this out with a simple math equation, 220 – (Your Age) = Your max heart rate. It is as simple as that, your max heart rate is the number of times that your heart can beat in a minute while your body is working at maximum exertion – working at max exertion is something that I strongly suggest for you not to try, only extreme athletes will work at this level as they have the training and experience.

You will use your max heart rate to work out what heart rate you should be working between. I will use the light training zone as an example here. So, I am 26 years old meaning that my max heart rate is 194bpm (220-26=194). To find the lower percentage of the training zone (60% for the light zone) you will have to do divide your max heart rate by 100 and times that new number by 60 (194 / 100 = 1.94 X 60 = 116.4 bpm), next you will do the same but times that number by 70 instead of 60 (194 / 100 = 1.94 X 70 = 135.8bpm). This means for me to work in between the light zone I will have to keep my heart rate between 116 bpm and 136bpm. I hope you understand how to use this to calculate other training zones.

**Progressive Overload**

Progressive overload is when the workload for a training session increases over time as the athlete adapts to training. Progressive overload is mainly used for strength training but can be used for helping with weight loss as well. If you decide to complete the same circuit 3 times a week for 6 weeks then yes you will get fitter, however you will not be able to get as fit as you could potentially be. For example, if an experienced athlete and a complete beginner both went into a room and completed 30 jumping jacks under the same conditions then the beginner will have a higher heart rate than the athlete as the athlete's body has adapted to exercise over all the years of training – therefore the athlete would have to work harder to get to the same heart rate as the beginner.

That should give you the idea that if you become fitter while training the same circuit then you will have to make it harder, if you just continue to train the exact same circuit then you will notice that your heart rate will gradually get lower each week while training. Progressive overload is the action of making the workouts harder each week so that you maintain the heart rate you need to work at. Working at the same heart rate will increase the rate of you losing weight. Below will be a short example of how you can implement progressive overload in circuits over time.

Week 1 - (Train Example Circuit 1) – Rest for 30 seconds between each exercise, complete 2 sets with a 3-minute rest between each set. Train at 60% of Max HR.

Warmup

1. Jumping Jacks – 30 seconds
2. Pushup – 30 seconds
3. Sit-ups – 30 seconds
4. Heel Flicks on Spot – 30 seconds

Cooldown

Week 2 - (Train Modified Example Circuit 1) – Rest for 30 seconds between exercises, complete 2 sets with a 3-minute rest between each set. Train at 60% of Max HR.

Warmup

1. Jumping Jacks – 45 seconds
2. Pushups – 45 seconds
3. Sit-ups – 45 seconds
4. Heel Flicks on Spot – 45 seconds

Cooldown

The six-week plan does not look like that as writing out the circuit for every day you are training would double the length of the book and I would rather get all the information over to you in the shortest book possible. But as you can see for the second week the exercises are 45 seconds long, this makes it harder than the first circuit as the exercises are only 30 seconds. Remember that is just an example just to show you how it works, in the six-week plan the progressive overload instructions are clear and easy to follow.

**Injury Prevention**

Injuries must be avoided at all costs. There are many injuries that you can get from training – the most common injuries for beginners are muscle strains. As your coach I want you to avoid all injuries at all costs. Injury can be very painful and may require hospital time if serious – I don't want you to experience pain and certainly have to spend time in hospital which may cost money for people in other countries. Injury is also a setback, you cannot train while injured for obvious reasons – this will stop your routine of training and losing weight.

Ways to Prevent Injury:
- Have the correct diet – Look at the diet section of this book for a refresh on what you should be eating and drinking. Your muscles need the energy to contract repeatedly during exercise. Consuming too much food every day would increase your chance of vomiting as the excess food isn't being used as energy it is just sat in the stomach weighing you down, not eating enough will put your body into a catabolic

state meaning that your body will be unable to properly repair tissue damage.

- Warming up before exercise. If you go straight into a hard workout then your muscles will be tight and more likely to strain if overstretched during exercise.

- Cooling Down after exercise – you need to allow your body to recover slowly.

- Have rest days – As a beginner, you should certainly not try to exercise every day as your body will not be used to it and you will be likely to pick up an injury. If you are getting started only exercise 3 or 4 times a week.

- Don't Train Through Pain – If you encounter pain while exercising then you are likely to have picked up an injury, do not continue to train as you will make the injury worse.

- Improve Flexibility – If your muscles have an extended range of motion that means it will be harder for them to get strained or pulled – the usual result of an injury. Stretching consistently will improve your flexibility, my circuits will also improve flexibility.
- Don't Train if Unwell – You will need to give your body time to recover from an illness as your body will constantly be working hard to fight away the illness. You may have low levels of energy when unwell making it difficult to train anyway.

If you feel like you have slight pain or injury just check with your doctor if you will be able to carry out the circuits provide. Now that I have covered all the important information, this is where the fun starts. The next chapter contains the circuits.

# Chapter 6 – The 5 Starter Circuits to Accelerate Weight Loss

Here is the part you have all been waiting for, this is the chapter that contains 5 circuits that can be done at home with no equipment. All you will need is a bit of open space and maybe a fitness mat to stop the floor from getting sweaty, don't exercise around furniture or valuable items just in case something gets broken, or you trip over.

I assume that you are overweight, and you have little experience when it comes to exercising. That is not a problem as that will change. I will have 2 very low impact circuits, 2 low impact circuits and a medium impact circuit that you can follow depending on your level. As a personal trainer, I am used to having the client right in front of me so I can coach them based on the ability they can show me, in this instance I cannot see what ability you are at. That's why this book has lots of variety within the exercises and intensity. Every exercise will be explained with a photo to show the demonstration in chapter 8.

You can mix and match the exercises from different circuits to make it suit you, as long as you follow a fitness routine then you are taking a step in the right direction to lose weight. The circuits will work out the entire body so that the weight loss will be much more noticeable. Work at the best level for you and do your best!

**Stretches**

Just before you get into the circuits, I am aware that as beginners you are more likely to have problems that restrict you from exercising to the best of your ability. The most common are joint issues which won't allow you to complete floor or low exercises with comfort, I want to offer common stretches and exercises that you can perform every day to strengthen your weak points so that you are ready to exercise. This isn't an alternative to the warmups, this is for those who struggle with the circuits.

Below is a list of stretches, each stretch will show which part of the body it targets and how it helps strengthens the joints. Hold these stretches for as long as you can, each day you stretch you should hopefully feel stronger in certain joints and more flexible.

**Lunges** – This stretch will strengthen your knees. These lunges will be slightly different from lunges that are included as an exercise in circuits throughout the circuits, these lunges are slower so that the quadriceps, hamstrings, calves, glutes are all strengthened which will make your knees and ankles stronger. To do a stretching lunge start by standing with legs shoulder-width apart, then take a big step with your left foot forwards and bend your knees into it, you will feel the stretch and hold this stretch for 10-15 seconds before stepping back and swapping legs. Place a hand on the floor to help you balance if needed, the photos below should help you find the form.

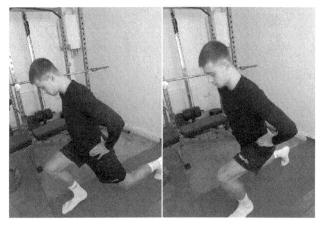

**Hip Swings** – This will allow you to have extended motion in your hips which prevents stiffness and pain. How to complete: Stand in an open space next to a wall, chair or something that can support your balance. Make sure that the open space is in front and behind you because you need to slowly swing your left leg forwards and back for around 30 seconds while keeping your other foot planted on the floor, remember to switch legs afterward and do the same for 30 seconds with the other leg.

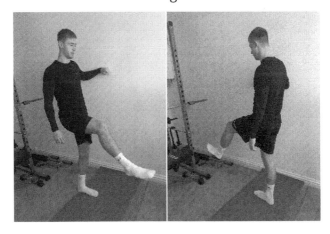

**Quadricep Stretch** – The benefits of stretching quads are that it helps you maintain balance, keeps your legs strong and decreases the chance of injury. You can discover how to stretch your quads in chapter 8 under the warmup exercise descriptions. The only difference is that you should hold the stretch for longer if you are trying to build up strength.

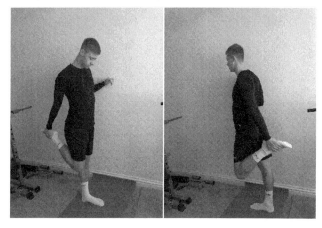

**Shoulder Roll**s – Improves range of mobility in shoulders. How to do it: Stand straight with arms straight down your side, then roll then forwards 10 times and backward ten times like the photo shows below. You can use your arms to create momentum to make the shoulder roll. The photo is hard to show how to do it, but hopefully you get the hang of it.

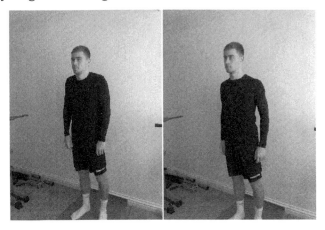

Try to complete these stretches every day so that you can build up the strength that will prepare you for the beginner circuits. If you are getting started and you feel like it is necessary for you to stretch every day for a couple of weeks before getting into the circuits then do it – you can use the two weeks to also fully focus on sorting out a healthy diet to follow in which you will hopefully be stuck to a healthy routine by the time you start training.

I suggest you spend 10 minutes a day on stretching, so split those stretches up whatever way suits you the most. Try not to push yourself too hard, these stretches should only be light. These stretches do not appear in the six-week plan, although lunges are involved in a circuit.

**Very Low Impact Circuit 1**

I recommend this to everyone as it is a good starting point to see where you are at. All the exercises in this circuit will be standing exercises, if you have joint problems then definitely stick to this circuit until you build up enough strength to move on. Remember, you and your doctor know your own body better than I do.

Complete circuit twice. Rest for 30 seconds in between each exercise and rest for 2 minutes after completing the first circuit. Train at Light Training Zone (Around 60% of Max HR). This circuit will last roughly 25 minutes including warmup and cooldown.

Warmup 1

1. Marching on the spot – 30 seconds
2. Half Lunges – 30 seconds
3. Hand Raises – 30 seconds
4. Side-to-side steps – 30 seconds
5. Hamstrings and rows – 30 seconds
6. Arm Circles – 30 seconds
7. Half Squat – 30 seconds
8. Knee Repeaters Left – 30 Seconds
9. Knee Repeaters Right – 30 seconds

Cooldown 1

**Very Low Impact Circuit 2**

The same difficulty as the first Very Low Impact Circuit, the difference being that some of the exercises are different to provide that variety. This also contains no floor exercises where you would need to bend low to complete meaning this will be easier to complete for those with joint problems.

Complete two sets. Rest for 30 seconds between each exercise. Rest for 2 minutes after completing the circuit then go again for the final set. Train at the light Training Zone (Around 60% of Max HR). This circuit will take roughly 30 minutes to complete including the warmup and cooldown.

Warmup 1
1. Marching on the Spot – 30 seconds
2. Shoulder Raise Half Lunge – 30 seconds

3. Open Gates – 30 seconds

4. High Knee and Backwards Kick – 30 seconds

5. Straight Punches – 30 seconds

6. Body Twists – 30 seconds

7. Box Step – 30 seconds

8. Knees to Hands – 30 seconds

9. Side Lunges – 30 seconds

Cooldown 1

**Low Impact Circuit 1**

Now you are looking at the step up from very low impact circuits, these exercises require more muscle groups to work and they will be worked harder than previously.

Repeat the circuit twice. Rest for 30 seconds between each exercise and rest for 2 minutes after completing the first set then go again. Train at light training zone (Around 65% of

Max HR). This circuit will take roughly 25 minutes to complete including the warmup and cooldown.

Warmup 2
1. Bounce on the spot – 30 seconds
2. Knees to Chest – 30 seconds
3. Jumping Jacks – 30 seconds
4. Sidestep Squats – 30 seconds
5. Uppercuts – 30 seconds
6. Knee Pushups – 30 seconds
7. Up and Out – 30 seconds
8. Left Right Floor Tap – 30 seconds

Cooldown 1

## Low Impact Circuit 2

Repeat circuit 3 times. Rest for 30 seconds between each exercise and rest for 2 minutes between sets. Train at the light training zone (Roughly 65% of Max Heart Rate). This circuit will take just under 30 minutes to complete including the warmup and cooldown.

Warmup 2
1. Open the Gates – 30 seconds
2. Stage 2 Pushups – 30 Seconds
3. Ankle Taps – 30 Seconds
4. Double Sidesteps – 30 seconds
5. Plank – 30 seconds
6. Twist and Punch – 1 minute

Cooldown 1

**Medium Impact Circuit**

This is the hardest circuit in this book, if you are looking for harder circuits move on to the next book in this series. Not to worry as this circuit can still be done by beginners and can also be modified to suit you. There are two harder circuits in the Basic Circuit Training Bundle.

Complete 3 sets, rest for 30 seconds between each exercise. Rest for 2 minutes after each set. Train at the moderate training zone (Around 70% of Max HR). This circuit will take roughly 30 minutes to complete including the warmup and cooldown.

Warmup 2
1. Jogging on the Spot – 30 seconds
2. Russian Twists – 30 seconds
3. Lunges with twists – 30 seconds
4. Straight Punches – 30 seconds
5. Lying Superman Hold – 30 seconds
6. Tuck Jumps – 30 seconds
7. Crunches – 30 seconds
8. Squats – 30 seconds

Cooldown 1

## How often to train

Before I waffle on, the next chapter contains a six-week plan which will sort out your diet and training routine for the next 6 weeks. Now that's out the way, I can show you how often you can train these circuits if you decide not to follow the six-week plan.

If you are a complete beginner then you will want to train 3 times a week with the very low impact circuits, gradually over a few weeks you will want to be able to complete 4 circuits a week. Start by training Monday, Wednesday, Friday. You will not need to train more than 4 times a week until you reach a level where you are comfortable to do so, you are the only person who knows when they are ready to make things harder. Ideally, I want everyone to work towards training for 30 minutes five times a week – this will meet the weekly recommended requirement of 150 minutes plus you will certainly be in good shape. I am not expecting you to get to that stage after a few weeks, that's why my follow up books will help you achieve this goal.

.

# Chapter 7 – The 6 Week Workout Routine

I have seen many people transform their bodies in six weeks and you are about to do the same thing. You will now go through the six-week plan, it is easy to follow and can will allow you to progress your fitness levels. The plan is clear to show where progressive overload has been used, what days to train and not train, with an overview of each week which will remind you to track progress. You are not to stop training after the six-weeks, this is to get you started in a routine and you can carry on towards your goals afterward by purchasing the next book or continuing with your own version.

First of all, I ask you to start this routine on a Monday, no better way to start the week. From this Monday you will **not** break your new diet and you **will** stick to your training routine. It's your job now to put in the work and watch it pay off. If you don't feel you are ready for this six-week plan, then remember to stretch every day and try to complete a very low impact circuit a few times before getting into this. Build yourself up to it.

**Six-Week Training Plan (Week 1 – The Start)**

Please train on the days it tells you to because it allows time for rest and recovery. For when you train on the day is completely up to you – I suggest you pick a time between two meals so you will have sufficient energy for it. I usually train after dinner and I make sure I have a snack for after the workout. That applies for all the weeks! Also, double-check which circuit to train as I have realized it is very easy to mix up "Very Low Impact Circuit 1" and "Low Impact Circuit 1".

**Monday –**

What to Train: Complete the Very Low Impact Circuit 1 as normal. (Complete to the best of your ability)

Progressive Overload Changes: None as it is just the first week.

**Tuesday –** Rest Day. Remember to try some of the recovery tips I listed earlier, this will prepare you for tomorrow's session.

**Wednesday –**

What to Train: Complete Very Low Impact Circuit 2 as normal

Progressive Overload Changes: This circuit is slightly harder but no changes to the actual circuits.

**Thursday –** Rest Day

**Friday -**

What to Train: Complete Very Low Impact Circuit 1.

Progressive Overload Changes: No changes. Try to see if you can complete more reps of certain exercises in the 30 second periods.

**Saturday** – Rest Day.

**Sunday** – Rest Day. Great work for this week, now it's time to get onto week 2.

**Week 1 overview:**

You shouldn't have found this extremely difficult, but if you did don't worry - all I suggest you repeat this week until you feel comfortable with going on the next week. You would have completed 85+ minutes of moderate exercise. Will increase this over time so you work towards the recommended 150 minutes of activity. No progressive overload changes yet.

**Week 2**

**Monday –**

What to Train: Complete Very Low Impact Circuit 2.

Progressive Overload Changes: Just like last Friday, try to complete more reps in the 30-second exercise period but this is just a suggestion.

**Tuesday –** Rest Day

**Wednesday –**

What to Train: Complete Low Impact Circuit 1

Progressive Overload Changes: As this is a harder circuit please complete this to the best of your ability with no changes.

**Thursday –** Rest Day

**Friday –**

What to Train: Complete Very Low Impact Circuit 1

Progressive Overload Changes: This is easier than low impact circuits, so this time spend 40 seconds on each exercise and keep every other variable the same. This will slightly increase the time you spend exercise making you burn more fat.

**Saturday –** Rest Day

**Sunday –** Rest Day. Cracking Stuff. Hope you are working well and most importantly getting it done at your own pace – onto week 3!

**Week 2 Overview:**

This week should be a slight step up from the first week. I include a new circuit into the plan "Low Impact Circuit 1", this is a slightly harder circuit than the very low impact circuits. I also increase the exercise period in the very low impact circuit 1 to make it harder. You would have completed 90+ minutes of exercise this week.

**Week 3**

**Monday –**

What to Train: Complete Low Impact Circuit 2

Progressive Overload Changes: None to this circuit, train this as normal.

**Tuesday –** Rest Day

**Wednesday –**

What to Train: Complete Very Low Impact Circuit 2

Progressive Overload Changes: Again, spend 40 seconds on each exercise with 30 seconds rest to increase the time that your heart is pumping quickly for.

**Thursday –** Rest Day

**Friday –**

What to Train: Complete Low Impact Circuit 1

Progressive Overload Changes: No new Changes to this circuit.

**Saturday –**

What to Train: Complete Low Impact Circuit 2

Progressive Overload Changes: No changes to the circuit, but you should notice an extra day of training for this week and the weeks to come.

**Sunday –** Rest Day. But today I urge you to try water therapy from the Rest and Recovery section because of the extra training load.

**Week 3 Overview:**

This week is a bigger step up with the difficulty to implement progressive overload, this is because you will be training 4 times a week from now on. This adds up to roughly 115+ minutes of moderate exercise every week, well on the way to meeting the recommended 150 minutes of recommended exercise each week. I also introduce Low Impact Circuit 2 this week, get used to it!

**Week 4**

**Monday –**
What to Train: Complete Very Low Impact Circuit 1

Progressive Overload Changes: Lower the resting time from 30 seconds between each exercise to 20 seconds, make sure you allow proper rest in this period as it now starts to get tough.

**Tuesday –** Rest Day

**Wednesday –**

What to Train: Complete Low Impact Circuit 1

Progressive Overload Changes: Spend 40 seconds on each exercise, just like how you do for the very-low impact circuits.

**Thursday –** Rest Day

**Friday –**

What to Train: Very Low Impact Circuit 2

Progressive Overload Changes: Lower the resting time from 30 seconds between each exercise to 20 seconds.

**Saturday –**

What to Train: Low Impact Circuit 2

Progressive Overload Changes: Increase the time spent on each exercise by 10 seconds, meaning you exercise for 40, rest for 30.

**Sunday –** Rest Day

## Week 4 Overview:

This week I made the circuits harder to complete by reducing the rest time on the very low impact circuits and for the low impact circuits, I increased the exercise periods. The weekly exercise duration will be a few minutes less than last week as I reduced the rest period – so around 110+ minutes of exercise for the week.

## Week 5

**Monday –**

What to Train: Low Impact Circuit 1

Progressive Overload Changes: No new changes from last week – keep it up!

**Tuesday –** Rest Day

**Wednesday –**

What to Train: Low Impact Circuit 2

Progressive Overload Changes: No new changes from last week. Still exercise for 40 seconds each time.

**Thursday –** Rest Day

**Friday –**

What to Train: Low Impact Circuit 1

Progressive Overload Changes: Complete Circuit in moderate training zone (Around 70% of max heart rate). This requires you to work harder during each exercise, you can do this by completing more reps of the certain exercise in the same 40 second period.

**Saturday –** Rest Day

What to Train: Low Impact Circuit 2

Progressive Overload Changes: Complete at 70% of Max HR like the other Low Impact Circuit.

**Sunday –** Rest Day

**Week 5 Overview:**

     For this week, I have stopped putting the very low impact circuits in the plan as I feel that these won't provide a real challenge to you unless modified to a large extent. However, I did modify the Low Impact Circuits by asking you to complete the circuits at 70% of your Max HR. You will get a sweat on for 110+ minutes this week.

**Week 6 – Final Week**

**Monday –**

What to Train: Low Impact Circuit 1

Progressive Overload Changes: Continue to work in the moderate training zone, the new addition will be that you should lower the rest period from 30 seconds to 20 seconds. The rest period between sets will stay the same.

**Tuesday –** Rest Day

**Wednesday –**

What to Train: Low Impact Circuit 2

Progressive Overload Changes: Continue to work in the moderate training zone, just reduce the resting duration to 20 seconds like the other low impact circuit.

**Thursday –** Rest Day

**Friday –**

What to Train: Medium-Impact Circuit

Progressive Overload Changes: Complete this circuit normally, this is a reasonably difficult circuit so do your best.

**Saturday –**

What to Train: Low Impact Circuit 1

Progressive Overload: No new changes, train this exactly like you trained on Monday. See this as a slight recovery session.

**Sunday –** Rest Day. The last day of the six-week plan but not your last day of training.

**Week 6 Overview:**

Firstly, I want to congratulate you on getting this far. It is a real achievement to try something new and stick to it. I hope that you notice positive changes with your body and you are in a great training routine now of exercising 4 times a week. So well done, I am proud of you. Remember to contact me or the Facebook group for additional help.

This is the only week where I introduce the medium impact circuit, this is a harder circuit so that is one of the ways I have implemented progressive overload. Another way I increased the difficulty was by increasing the length of the exercise period – this also means you exercise roughly 115+ minutes a week.

Although this is the final week, this doesn't mean that you stop after this week. You can continue to train by looking at how I have made the plan and how I made it harder. Or you can crack onto my second book of the series that will pick it up from this moment. How you train is up to you, as long as you stick to it and see the results then I have no problem. I suggest working your way towards training 5 times a week or getting to 150 minutes of moderate exercise each week.

# Chapter 8 – How to Complete Every Exercise for the Circuits

No messing around, I will list each exercise and explain it in this chapter. Some may have photo examples to help you get the correct form. The form is very important because if you do not complete reps for certain exercises correctly then it is likely you will pick up an injury. Check out @dec.beales on Instagram, I would like to thank him for demonstrating all of the exercises for me.

For the majority of the exercises, I start by describing the starting position, the picture for that is below. That is what I mean by standing straight with feet shoulder-width apart. This will not apply to the floor exercises.

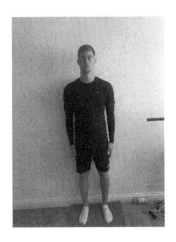

**Very Low Impact Exercises**

**Marching on the spot** – Stand straight with feet shoulder-width apart. Start on your left leg by raising your left knee and right arm. Raise your leg to a point where you feel comfortable, then, lower your right arm and left leg so you can repeat on the alternative side. The photos below should help, marching should be done in a smooth motion. This exercise is light but gets you moving and your heart pumping.

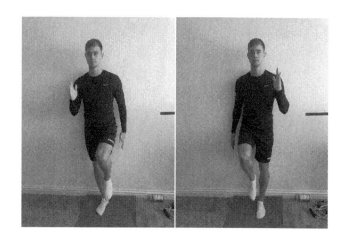

**Half Lunges –** This is the easier version of lunges. Stand straight to start, step out with your left foot and place it down, facing forwards. Keep your right foot planted then slightly bend both knees and place your weight onto your front leg. Hold that position for a second or two before stepping back with your left foot and repeating with your right leg. Alternate sides for 30 seconds. This exercise strengthens your legs (Quads and Calves) and will get the blood pumping around your body.

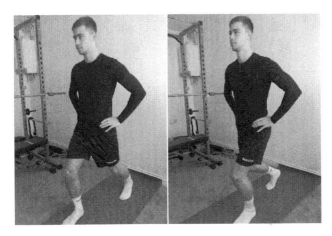

**Hand Raises** – Start in the normal standing position and hold your hands out to the side like shown in the left picture. Then raise your hands as high as possible (shown in the right picture), once in that position, lower your hands back to the starting position and continue to raise and lower your hands. Continue to repeat this for 30 seconds and feel free to march on the spot at the same time if you find this too easy.

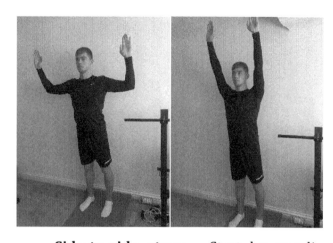

**Side-to-side steps** – Start by standing straight with feet apart. Firstly take a step to the right with your right foot and slightly bend your knees into it(the 3rd picture shows this), from the right step position step to the left with your right foot and place your foot next to your left foot(2nd picture), then step left with your left foot and bend your knees into it like the 1st photo shows. Once you get into the rhythm it will become natural and is a real fun cardiovascular exercise. Repeat this for 30 seconds by going from right to left, then left to right and so on…

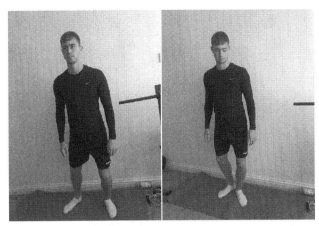

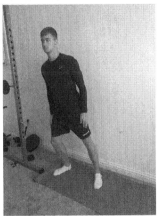

**Hamstring and Rows** - The pictures should help you with this. Stand straight, keep arms down in front of you - pretend that you are holding onto a pole with your hands. Pull up as if you are rowing a boat, at the same time kick your left leg back so your heel is flicked towards your bum. Then lower your left foot to the floor while pushing down with your hands back to the starting position and repeat with your right foot. Continue this left-right-left movement for 30 seconds. This is a fun exercise to strengthen your legs and get you sweating.

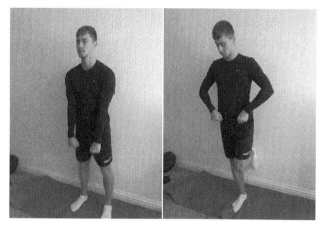

**Arm Circles** – Start by standing tall and bring your arms out straight on either side so that you are shaped like a capital "T". Imagine that you are drawing circles with your fingers, start by drawing small circles then slowly make your circles bigger.

You will be using your shoulders to get the circular motion in your arms, switch direction after 15 seconds. You can choose how small or big you draw your circles as long as you keep them rotating. The pictures below should help, from isn't all too important as long as you are rolling your shoulders to reduce stiffness in your upper body.

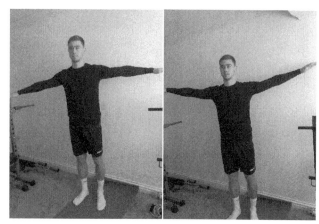

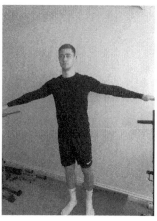

**Half Squat** - Start with feet shoulder-width apart and slightly turned outwards. Put weight into your heels, sit your bum back and bend your knees slightly until you get to a position which the 2nd picture shows, afterwards push up with your legs to stand back in the starting position. Don't bend knees too much for this level as you may find it painful when getting back up. You can put your arms out in front of you like the photos shows for balance support. You should keep squatting down and pushing up for 30 seconds, will increase muscle mass in your legs as it works your calves, hamstrings, glutes and quads.

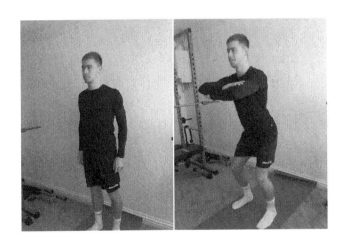

**Knee Repeaters Left -** Start by standing in a half lunge position in which your left foot is placed much further back than your right foot. Keep both legs slightly bent and hold your hands out in front like the 1st photo shows below. Then bring your left knee to your hands and after they connect place your foot back in the starting position. Your right foot should stay planted while you continuously move your left knee forwards and back for 30 seconds. This exercise is great for improving your balance, flexibility in your hips and mainly strengthens your core. Apologies about the angles of the photos, they both work the same leg.

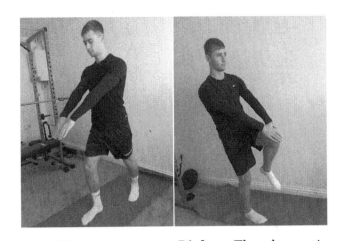

**Knee Repeaters Right** – The alternative to Knee Repeaters Left. Start by standing in a half lunge position but have your right foot placed much further back than your left foot. Then bring your right knee to where you hold your hands out in front, once they connect place your right foot back in the starting position. Remember to keep your left foot planted and repeat for 30 seconds. This has the same benefits as "knee repeaters left". Both exercises should be included in the same circuit if you are making your own to provide balance. Sorry about the angle again.

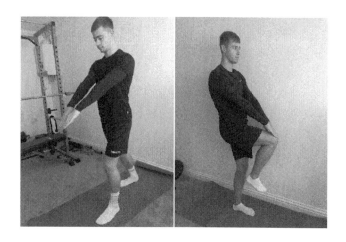

**Very Low Impact Circuit 2 Exercises**

**Shoulder Raise Half Lunge** – This is a combination of hand raises and half lunges. Start in the usual standing position, with hands up by your side like you're surrendering (2nd photo). Of course, you're not going to surrender because you should step backward with your left foot and at the same time raise both your arms up either side of you as far up as possible (3rd photo). Hold for a second before stepping your left foot back into the starting position and lowering your arms. Then step back with your right foot while raising your arms (1st photo), finally step forwards into the starting position and lower arms. Repeat this for 30 seconds, remember to swap legs each time. This exercise will improve your overall coordination and will work major muscles in arms and legs.

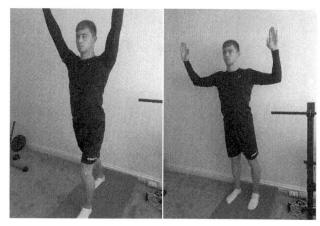

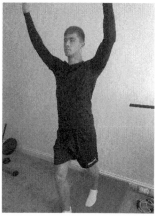

**Open Gates -** Start in the casual starting position. Lead with your left leg, imagine you are drawing the letter 'n' to your left. Do that by raising your left knee in front of you then twist your hip to rotate your leg 90 degrees to the left and then lower your leg. Repeat this on the right side. The photos below will help your form, switch legs every time you open the gate and repeat for the time given. Will reduce stiffness in your hips/groin and improve balance.

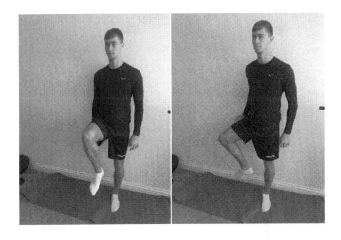

**Straight Punches** – Start by standing in a causal boxing stance, do this by placing your weak foot (pointing forwards) in front of your strong foot (facing outwards) with your arms held high and fists clenched like the 1st photo shows below

– always keep your knees slightly bent. To throw a left straight punch then simply extend your left arm out quickly until you cannot extend your arm anymore, which then you should instantly bring your arm back to the starting position – always keep a clenched fist and the punch should be like a snap. To throw a right straight punch, follow the same steps as the left straight punch but twist your body while the punch is thrown. My boxing book can always help you with form. The benefits from this include faster hands, will make you sweat and potentially hand eye coordination. Repeat left-right-left-right straight punches for the time period.

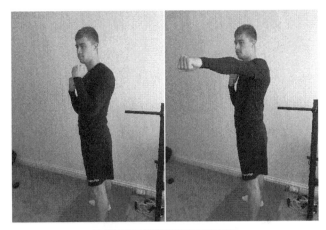

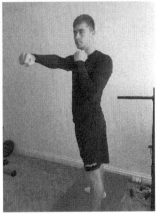

**Body Twists** – Start by standing with knees slightly bent and feet shoulder-width apart. Hold your hands together in front of your torso. Keep your feet planted on the ground, then use your arms and lower back to twist your body slowly from side to side. Repeat that motion for the time given. This exercise is great for strengthening your abs/core, lower back and improving flexibility.

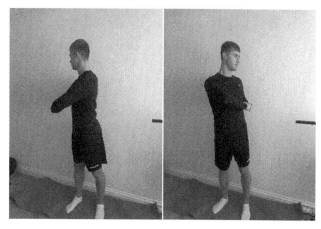

**Box Steps** – Stand with feet slightly wider than shoulder-width apart. Then from that position step forwards with your left foot while keeping your knees slightly bent (1st photo), then step forwards with your right foot so you are in a sort of half squat position (photo 2), then step back with your left foot followed by your right foot to get back to the starting position. Practice the steps slowly until you get into rhythm, once you get the hang of it exercise in the circuits for the time given. This exercise is good for strengthening leg muscles.

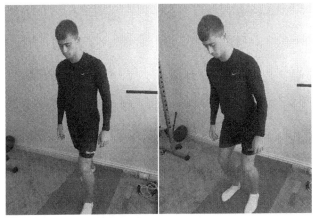

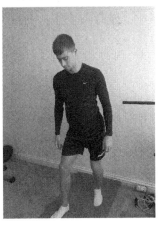

**Knees to hands** – Stand straight with feet slightly wider than shoulder-width apart. Hold both hands out straight in front of you as shown below. Then raise your left knee to your right hand and lower it back to starting position after touching. After you have lowered your left leg, raise your right knee to your left hand then lower your right leg after they connect. Will be like a crisscross. Carry this exercise out for time given, great for burning belly fat, improving balance and strengthening obliques.

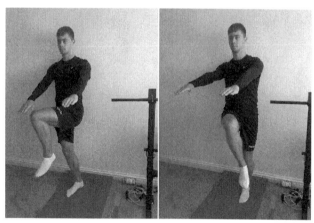

**Side Lunges-** Begin by standing light on your feet with feet slightly apart. Lunge left by stepping as far as you can left with your left foot and bend your left knee into it. Keep your right leg straight, your feet should always face outwards and always face forwards. From that position keep your feet planted to the ground, lean to the right side and switch your legs so that your left leg is now straight and your right leg is bent. Continue to switch from side to side, this exercise will work your core, quads and glutes. The pictures below should help.

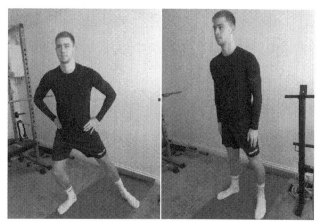

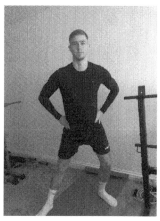

**Low Impact Exercises**

    **Bouncing on the spot** – Very simple. Stand normally with feet shoulder-width apart and stand on your tiptoes. Then press up and down repeatedly with your tiptoes so that you are bouncing slightly. Try not to let your heels touch the floor. No photo provided due to the simplicity of it.

**Knees to chest (Floor)** – Lay on the floor facing the ceiling. In one motion: Bring your knees up towards your chest using your hips and core, then hold onto your legs like the 2nd photo shows for a couple of seconds before letting go and returning to the laying-down position. Continue that movement for the time allocated for exercise. Make sure you use your core to get your knees up and this exercise is brilliant for improving flexibility and core strength.

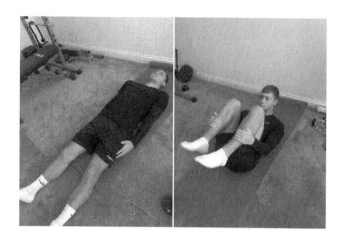

**Jumping Jacks** – Start standing with feet together and arms down by your sides (Photo 1). In one motion bend your knees and spring up into the air, separate your legs and raise your hands so your body is in a star shape. Land in the star shape (Photo 2) and from this position spring up again to get yourself back into the starting position by lowering your arms and closing legs. Repeat this motion, this exercise is very good for cardio which contributes towards burning calories and fat.

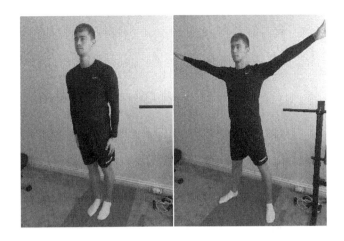

**Sidestep Squats** – Very similar to side to side steps. Start as normal and carry out the side to side steps. Every time you step to either side you need to slightly squat on the transition of stepping to the side, for example, if you are about to step to the left you will want to slightly bend your knees before you place your left foot on the ground. The pictures should help. This will work the main leg muscles, core and lower back. Sidestep squat from left to right, then right to left on repeat until done.

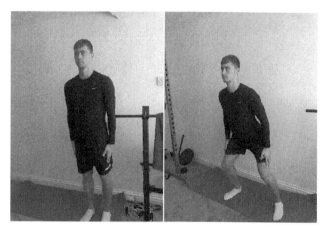

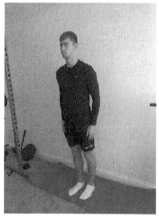

**Uppercuts** – Get into the causal boxer stance that I previously explained with the "Straight Punches" however you can keep your guard lower. Punch up in the air with both arms in the order of left-right-left-right, you will need to lower your arm after every punch so you can punch again. The form is not that important for this instance, but you will get a sweat on. Try not to punch too high, if you are looking to into a mirror then your punches should stop around your chin.

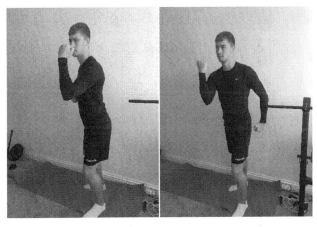

**Knee Pushups**- Place both knees on the floor and your hands on the floor so that your body is kept off the floor. From this position lower your chest to the ground by bending your elbows, once your chest is close to the ground use your arms to push up back to the starting position. Continue to lower and raise your chest using your arms for the time given, having your knees on the ground makes this exercise easier because you will have less of your body weight to push up. Will strengthen your triceps, pectorals and shoulders as well as maintaining your higher heart rate.

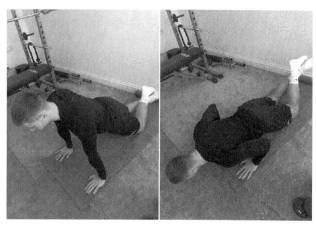

**Up and Out** – Start in the usual standing position. Start on the left side by stepping to the left while extending your arm to the left and point your finger like the 1st photo shows, from that position bring your left foot forwards and bring your left hand to the sky (2nd photo). Keep your right foot planted in the same position for the entire time. Repeat these steps alternatively for the right side, it may look like you're dancing in the sixties. Just a fun cardiovascular exercise.

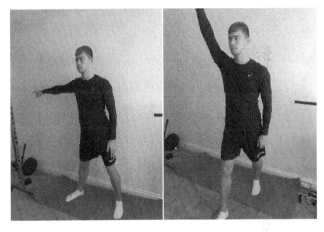

**Left Right Floor Tap** – Begin by standing with legs slightly bent and your hands down by your sides. Reach down with your left hand and tap the floor to the left of your left foot, stand back up and repeat this but tap with your right hand to the right side of your right foot. Continue this motion for the time given. Remember to bend your legs when bending down to avoid back injuries. Strengthens lower back.

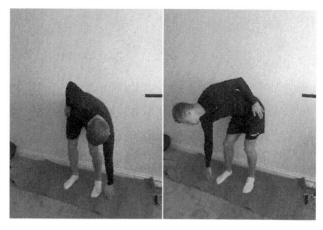

**Low Impact Circuit 2**

**Open the gates** – Previously Explained, description found under the "Very Low Impact Exercises".

**Ankle Taps** – Begin by laying down on the floor facing the sky. Keep your arms by your sides as you need to mainly use your arms in this exercise. Your feet should be planted on the floor. To complete an ankle tap: Reach for your left ankle with your left hand and try to tape your ankle, remember to stay in the initial laying position. Afterwards, bring your left hand back while reaching out to tap to your right ankle with your right hand. This exercise is great for strengthening obliques. Continue to tap both ankles for the time given.

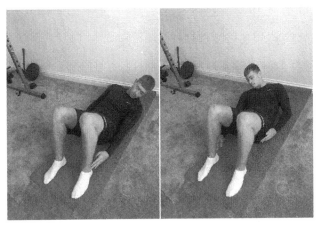

**Double Sidestep-** (Make sure you have plenty of space) This is just a sidestep which is previously explained, the difference being you are required to sidestep in each direction twice before switching direction. For example, from the starting standing position you will step left with your left foot, bring your right foot across and then step left again before switching direction. This is a fun cardio exercise which will improve your agility. No photos provided as it would look just like a normal sidestep.

**Plank-** Begin by laying on the floor facing the floor and keep your forearms flat on the ground underneath your chest along with the rest of your body. To get into the plank push up slightly with your forearms and your feet so that the only parts of your body connecting with the floor are your arms and tiptoes. Hold this position for the time given if you can, feel free to go onto your knees if you find this too difficult. This exercise is fantastic for our entire body, but most importantly burns belly fat and builds up abs. The photo below shows the plank in action, don't raise your bum too high while planking as that is cheating, you should feel the burn.

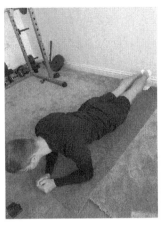

**Twist and Punch** – Begin in the position that picture 1 shows, to do this place your left foot in front of your right and point it forwards, extend your arm out in front of you with your fist clenched and your right foot should be back at a 90 degrees angle to the right so that you're stood side on. To get to the stance of picture 2, step back with your left foot so that its pointing to the left while bringing your fist back to your chest, then step forwards with your right foot and extend your right arm like you are punching. Continue to switch stances for the time given, will improve coordination and get you sweating.

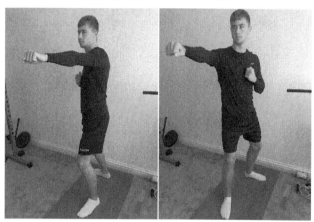

**Medium Impact Exercises**

**Jogging on the Spot** – Light run on the spot, just transfer weight from one leg to the other repeatedly. No picture included, c'mon everyone knows how to jog on the spot.

**Russian Twists** - Start in a sitting position so that your body and upper legs are in a "V" shape, to do this sit up on the floor while slightly leaning back, have your knees slightly raised and bent (1st photo). Start on the left side by holding your hands together next to your left hip, use your core and lower back to twist your body from left to right and use your hands to tap the floor either side of your body. Tap from left to right, right to left for the time given. Cross your ankles if you feel it help you balance. This exercise strengthens obliques, abs and lower back.

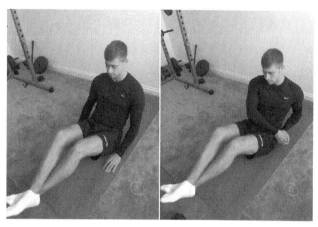

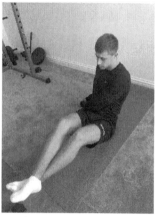

**Lunges with twists-** The lunge has already been described as a stretch in this book, however there are 2 differences. The first difference is that you will not hold the lunge for as long as you would if you were stretching.

Secondly, every time you lunge forwards, your will use your lower back and arms to twist your body left then right before standing back up in the starting position. This exercise is almost an entire body workout that improve balance, flexibility and strengthens your lower body.

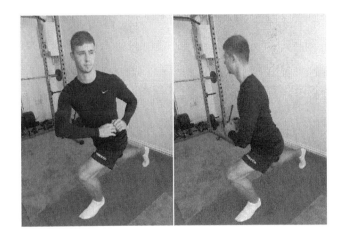

**Straight Punches** – This has been previously explained as a very low impact exercise, the only difference is that you will be throwing the punches slightly faster to keep your heart rate at the moderate training zone.

**Lying Superman Hold** – Starting position: Picture 1 shows that you should lay down facing the floor with your arms slightly in front of you bent and your legs slightly apart while relaxed. Then use your core and back to raise your arms and legs off the ground, hold this position for a second or two before relaxing your muscles back into the starting position. Continue this for 30 seconds, a great core exercise.

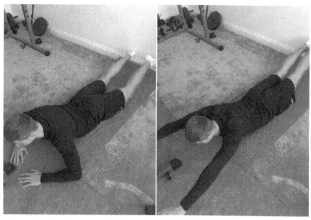

**Tuck Jumps** – From the usual standing position bend your knees slightly and push through your heels to jump up into the air, once your feet have left the ground tuck your knees into your chest by bending them. Be careful as you need to prepare for the impact of your fall so don't spend too long in the tuck position. This exercise will build up power in your leg muscles, along with help you burn fat and allow you to get worn out quickly. Don't worry about trying to jump as high as dec here!

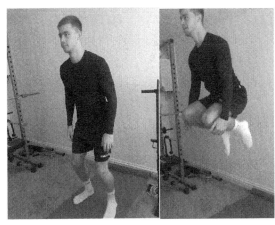

**Crunches** – Start by laying on the floor facing the sky with your arms crossed over your chest. Bring your knees up and make sure your feet are together while planted on the floor. From this starting position use your core and lower back to bring your chest about halfway to your knees, once you reach this point slowly release and lower yourself back to the ground. Complete as many as you can in the time, this will let you build up abs and burn belly fat.

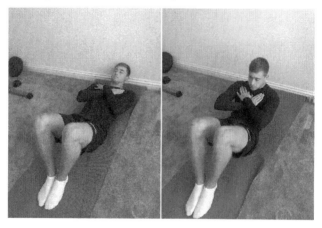

**Squats** –Start with feet shoulder-width apart and pointing outwards. Put weight into your heels, sit your bum back and bend your knees to lower yourself until your thighs are almost parallel to the floor, from this position push up through your heels to complete a squat. Keep your arms out in front of you while doing this to improve balance and avoid this exercise if you have knee problems. This exercise is brilliant for building stronger legs.

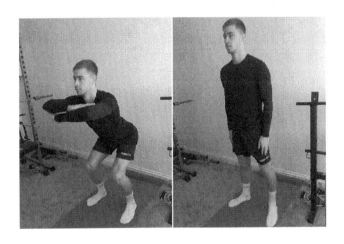

I have now described every exercise used in this book. More Exercises and Descriptions are available in my other books or the Basic Circuit

Training Bundle. More descriptions are below for the Warmup and Cooldown exercises.

## Warmup Exercise Descriptions

**Walking on the spot** – Self-explanatory. Pretend you're walking slowly by lifting and lowering your left leg then right reg, feel free to actually walk around if you have space for it.

**Arm Swings** – Start with arms by your side and simply swing both arms up as high as you can and back down again. Keep swinging for 30 seconds.

**Overhead Triceps Stretch** – To stretch left arm: Lift left arm up straight and bend your elbow, reach as far down your back as you can with your left hand. Then push down on your left elbow with your right hand to stretch your triceps. Hold for 10 – 15 seconds then repeat with your right arm by completing the steps alternatively.

**Childs Pose** – This is great for your back. Get into a kneeling position and place hands on the floor in front of you. Then stretch your arms forwards by shuffling your hands across the floor. You will feel your lower back being stretched, hold this for as long as you can in 30 second period.

**Standing Hamstring Stretch** – To stretch left leg: Start by standing up straight, then bend your right knee slightly while extending your left leg so your left heel is on the floor and your toes are pointing upwards. Hold this stretch for 10-15 seconds then switch leg by repeating steps alternatively. If you don't feel anything the press your hands above your knee on your bent leg as this force will certainly stretch the hamstrings.

**Marching on the spot** – Already described at the start of this chapter. March for 60 seconds.

**Arm circles** – Previously explained as an exercise, this time just move your arms slower in circles than normal.

**Left Right Floor Taps** – Find the description earlier on in this chapter. Complete at a very light intensity for 60 seconds.

**Quad Stretch** – This requires a good level of balance so try to get something sturdy to lean on. Start standing in the usual position. Bring your left heel to your bum and hold it there with your left hand, use your right hand to lean on a sturdy object and hold this for 10-15 seconds. Swap to your right leg afterward. Pictures for this are found under "Stretches" in chapter 6.

**Cross-body Shoulder Stretch** – Can be done standing or sitting. Start with your left shoulder: Bring your extended left arm across your torso so your left hand is past your right shoulder. With your right wrist, you want to press on your left wrist towards you so that you feel the burn in your left shoulder. Repeat this but follow the steps alternatively to stretch your right shoulder. Hold this for 10-15 seconds each arm.

**Chest Expansion** – Dynamic Stretch. Start by standing straight with your arms extended in front of you together like you have just clapped. Keep arms extended, separate your arms and bring them back as far as you can until your chest is puffed out. Hold that position for a second before bringing your arms forwards and your hands together. This should be done all in one motion, keep repeating for 30 seconds.

**Cooldown Exercise Descriptions**

**Light March on Spot** – Just a slower version of marching on the spot, which I have already described.

**Close the Gates** – Start by standing in the usual position. Start with your left leg: Twist your body 90 degrees to the left and lift your left knee upwards, then rotate your hips to bring your knee parallel to your other knee and then bring your foot down. Switch legs and complete the steps but alternatively, do this for 30 seconds and if it helps it is the opposite movement to opening the gates. (A previously described exercise/stretch)

**Shoulder shrugs** – Can be done standing or sitting. Simple keep your arms down by the side of you and shrug your shoulders up and relax to bring them down. You can also roll your shoulders back to get an extra range of motion. Very similar to shoulder rolls, the only difference being is that you don't have to push your shoulders back to bring them down.

**Shake off the body** – Just get the blood flowing around the body by shaking your arms and legs. Do this how you like, there isn't really a correct form for it.

**Seated Spinal Twists** – Sit on the floor with a straight back. Simply just twist your body using your lower back to the left then right repeatedly but slowly. Use your arms to help twist your body. Do this for 30 seconds. This will improve flexibility in your lower back.

**Seated Hamstring Stretch** – Sit on the floor with back straight and legs extended. Reach forward with both hands and try to touch your toes while keeping legs straight, no worries if you can't touch your toes but just reach as far forwards as you can and hold it for 10 seconds and repeat that twice in the 30 second period.

# Chapter 9 – What's Next for Your Future of Fitness?

As you know, this book has a target audience for people who hardly exercise – it is hard for me to know the exact shape and size of the readers, but I will assume you are heavier than the average person. There is no problem with that as this particular book will slim you down to get out of the blob shape to a healthier shape.

After the six-week plan, I hope that you have made progress with weight loss so you can carry on to the next book – a next book you may ask?

"Intermediate Circuit Training", this is the sequel to this book that you are reading now. This next book will be able to take your training further by increasing the difficulty of the workouts, the strictness of the diets and more tips to help you get into the shape you want. I believe this book to also be very beneficially for readers mentally, reading the parts about mindset will hopefully change your outlook on your unhealthy lifestyle.

The final book of this series will be for getting into insane shape. I used HIIT styled circuits that will definitely get you into a defined shape. But you will have a long way to go from here.

Obviously, you don't have to buy my books. You can simply just continue to train how you are at the moment – whether you use my help or not is up to you. I just hope that my message has got across to you – Please stay in a training routine because once you fall out of a routine it is much harder to get back into one. Remember, some exercise is better than no exercise and 2 cheat meals is better than 7 cheat meals a week.

# Conclusion

Thank you for making it to the end of Circuit Training for beginners! I hope that you enjoyed this book, and you can take the information to help you reach your fitness goals. Remember that losing weight is not a race, it's more of a marathon, so please take it at your own pace and stick to it. I would suggest your next step would be to carry on reading this series and getting straight into the second book "Intermediate Circuit Training".

This book covered the complete basics of exercising using circuit training. I started this book laying down some hard-hitting stats and facts about obesity and why the people who find themselves in an overweight/obese state should make a change. In the second chapter, I list the basics of circuit training including the variables, the benefits, an example circuit, an example week plan and the short list of equipment that can help you while training. In the third chapter, I talk about how important diet is when it comes to losing weight and helping you with training. Also, in this chapter I provide a week's diet plan that you can choose to follow. The diet plan is very broad because there are many people different shapes and sizes with different intolerances and what not so it would be very hard to make it specific while suiting everyone Chapter 4 is the chapter where I talk about how things outside of training like warmups, cooldowns, resting and recovering contribute to you getting the best results possible. Chapter 5 focuses on injury prevention, how to implement progressive overload and the training zones so you can work efficiently towards your goals.

Chapter 6 is where the fun starts as I list 5 circuits at different difficulties that you can do at home with no equipment – train how you like and you have the choice whether to participate in the six-week plan. There are many basic stretches in this chapter as well which can help you build up strength. That links nicely to chapter 7 where I have the six-week training plan laid out. Chapter 8 contains all the exercise descriptions, most of them including pictures which the amazing Dec Beales modelled. Chapter 9 is a short chapter that informs you to not stop and gives you the option to take your training further. That was a brief overview of the book to refresh your memories.

As a personal trainer, I find it much easier to train people 1 to 1 as I can see how they train and the progress they make. However, although writing allows me to reach more people, I sadly cannot see who I am training so that's why I cannot aim this book for people at a certain weight and whatnot. I hope that I have helped in some way and if you read this and feel like it doesn't work for you then no worries – at least you gave it a go.

My other two books on circuit training may also be helpful for you so please give them a read, it would mean everything. It is now up to you to push yourselves further and I support you in every step of the way.

Finally, if you found this book useful in any way then an honest review on this would be greatly appreciated. Feedback is greatly appreciated as it allows me to pass on information in the most effective way to help people reach their goals.

# References

*Dec Beales - Model for the Exercise*

*Demonstrations.*

https://www.instagram.com/dec.beales/

*Your Free Gift – The Circuit Training Weight Loss*

*Bundle.*

*https://hudsonandrew.activehosted.com/f/33*

*Join the Facebook Community.*

https://www.facebook.com/groups/workoutf

orweightloss

*Follow my Facebook Page.*

https://www.facebook.com/andrewhudsonbo

oks1

*Email me for extra support.*

andrew@hudsonandrew.com

*BMI calculator.* (n.d.). Patient.Info.

https://patient.info/doctor/bmi-calculator-calculator

*Recommended calorie intake.* (n.d.). Calculator.Net.

https://www.calculator.net/calorie-calculator.html

*Obesity problems.* (2019). NHS.

https://www.nhs.uk/conditions/obesity/#:~:text=Being%20obese%20can%20also%20increase,coronary%20heart%20disease%20and%20strok

Procon.org. (2016). *Global obesity population*.

Obesity.procon.

https://obesity.procon.org/global-obesity-levels/

M.L. (2019). *Training recovery*. Verywellfit.

https://www.verywellfit.com/ways-to-speed-recovery-after-exercise-3120085

J. (2017). *Healthy lifestyle benefits*. Themarlowclub.

https://themarlowclub.co.uk/top-ten-benefits-to-keeping-fit-and-healthy/

*Why circuit training?* (n.d.). Miamiathleticclub.

https://www.miamiathleticclub.org/stories-news/fitness/why-circuit-training-5-reasons-to-use-it-in-your-workouts#:~:text=Circuit%20training%20is %20a%20high,for%20variety%20in%20you r%20workouts.

D.B. (2020). *Progressive overload.* Healthline. https://www.healthline.com/health/progressi ve-overload

*Injury prevention.* (2017). Healthychildren. https://www.healthychildren.org/English/hea lth-issues/injuries-emergencies/sports-injuries/Pages/Sports-Injuries-Treatment.aspx

Bodyproject. (n.d.). *Some circuit exercises (video).* Youtube.

https://www.youtube.com/c/BodyProjectcha
llenge

A. (2020a). *Floor exercises*. Stylesatlife.
https://stylesatlife.com/articles/floor-
exercises/

A.G. (2021). *Lunch ideas*. Goodhousekeeping.
https://www.goodhousekeeping.com/food-
recipes/healthy/g960/healthy-lunch-ideas/

M.L.C. (2020c). *Chicken + rice meals*. Delish.
https://www.delish.com/cooking/g177/chick
en-rice-recipes/

M.F. (2020c). *Healthy dinner ideas*. Delish.
https://www.delish.com/cooking/recipe-
ideas/g3733/healthy-dinner-recipes/

M.A. (2021b). *More healthy dinner ideas.*
Countryliving.
https://www.countryliving.com/food-
drinks/g4288/healthy-dinner-recipes/

F.S. (2019a). *Healthy snacks.* Healthline.
https://www.healthline.com/nutrition/29-
healthy-snacks-for-weight-
loss#TOC_TITLE_HDR_5

# Intermediate Circuit Training

*The Mistakes Most People Make When Trying to Lose Weight at Home and How to Avoid Them.*

**Andrew Hudson**

# Introduction

Having a goal is great. It gives you something to work towards which is often rewarding once the goal is reached. Not every goal that's set is fun every step of the way because people may find it too difficult, they haven't got the time for it or they aren't making any progress. A goal which is common for many people is weight loss because they are unhealthy, out of shape and not confident in their own body. Unfortunately, it doesn't always go to plan because for several reasons. The most common being that they follow poor workouts, have an unhealthy diet and have no mental strength to get things done.

You have a goal of losing weight, I know this because you are reading this book. There are many reasons why you want to lose weight, but you know that the outcome of you losing weight will benefits you and I am here to help you get to your fitness goal. This book is presented with simple nutritional advice and many workouts to get you into a healthy routine so that you don't just give up, instead you will reach your fitness goal.

Who am I? Just a qualified Personal Trainer with a few years of experience under the belt. Why should you take my advice? Because I take consideration of the restrictions that people face when it comes to exercising, I help people get around the restrictions so they can reach their goals. I have spent many long nights researching and writing these books to pass the information over in a motivational way as I know it isn't easy just to read a book and suddenly get into a fitness routine. Over the years, many people have thanked me for supporting them on their weight loss journey. I also benefit from this because it feels great to see the gradual progress made by people and the joy it brings to their life.

If you have a bit of a belly that you want to flatten, or if you want to drop down a couple of sizes, or if you want to look good for an event, if you haven't got enough money for a gym membership, if you can't afford gym equipment or finally if you are just simply bored of your current workout routine. Then carry-on reading. This book makes exercise simple, fun, quick and can be done at home – saving you time and money from going to the gym.

I will be using the training method Circuit Training to direct you towards your goals of losing weight. The circuits I provide require absolutely no equipment, but I do suggest some that are optional to help you succeed. This book provides 8 circuits that can be set up and completed quickly, a description of every exercise with a photo, dietary advice to help you lose weight more efficiently, plenty of motivation and much more that you can discover if you keep reading. This book isn't quite for the complete beginners, more for people who have a bit of experience with exercise. This book is the second of this series, so if you are looking for beginner workouts then lookout for Circuit Training for Beginners.

The "I will do it tomorrow" mindset is not the mindset that will allow you to reach your goals. With hard work comes great rewards and that is why you should get this book now. If you even just consider following this book, then you are already at a disadvantage. You need to fully commit, because if you follow the advice in this book then you will start to see positive changes to your body over time and put yourself in the best position possible to reach your fitness goals. So, are you keep sitting on that fence by saying you'll do it tomorrow? Believe me, I know what sitting on the fence is like and it brings me nothing more than regret.

**Circuit Training for Weight Loss**

This is the second book from the three-part series, "Circuit Training for Weight Loss". This series is for people that are looking to reach fitness goals at home with the training method: Circuit Training. Whether your goal is to lose weight to avoid health risks, to improve your health or if you are looking to lower your body fat percentage to look ripped/toned, then this series will help you out. Below you will find a brief description of each book and a summary of the series at the end, if you want to find out more, then search up the book titles to view the detailed description!

The first book of this series, "Circuit Training for Beginners", is the prequel to this book. This book is the most basic as it is for those who have a lower level of experience when it comes to health & fitness. This book will get you into a simple exercise routine, will help you clean up your diet and give you an understanding of general health and fitness. Making this book a great starting point to set you off on your weight loss journey, helping you break your old unhealthy habits so you can no longer fall under the obese or overweight category. I suggest for all beginners to read this first book before continuing with "Intermediate Circuit Training".

The book you are currently reading, "Intermediate Circuit Training", is a step up that increases the difficulty of the workouts, so you make quicker progress towards harder fitness goals. This still sticks with the theme of weight loss with circuit training and nutrition, but this book starts to branch out to slightly more advanced health & fitness information and starts to present motivational advice, so you stay on track with your fitness goal. This isn't for complete beginners, more for the average person looking to lose weight.

The final book, "High Intensity Circuit Training", is the most advanced book. The workouts in these books are shorter, but much more difficult and frequent as this book is to help people with difficult fitness goals like having a low body fat percentage and having a high lean muscle mass percentage. This book also offers advice on how to adapt your mindset to reach challenging goals, information about how to boost your metabolic rate and many other ways to burn fat quickly to lower your body fat percentage while building lean muscle mass. This is for the experienced fitness fanatics.

As you can see, each book from this series is like a steppingstone towards your final fitness goal. Each book goes up in difficulty and if you are looking to go from Fat to Fit, I highly recommend following each book 1 at a time to reach and maintain your goal of having your dream body!

# Your Free Gift

The gift is a free eBook titled - "The Circuit Training Weight Loss Bundle". In this bundle you will find some 'extras' that will help you lose weight quicker, such as:

- An equipment checklist that contains all the optional equipment listed in this book with a link to where you can buy the product for a reasonable price.

- Secondly, you will find a diet tracker – This allows you to plan out your diet for the week and track all the nutrients and calories you consume, planning saves time and money!

- A Training Plan that you can edit yourself to make it specific for you, this allows you to have your own routine that doesn't mess up any plan. Plus a few more things you will have to see for yourself by getting the eBook.

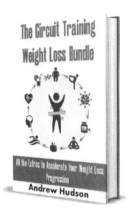

Follow this link to access the free eBook:

https://hudsonandrew.activehosted.com/f/33

# Join the Workout for Weight Loss Community

Living a healthy lifestyle is difficult, especially when you feel as if you are doing it all alone. That's why I suggest for you to join a community of others who are in your situation, this community "Workout for Weight Loss" will provide you with daily posts about weight loss and there will be many people that you can talk to, share experiences with and receive help from.

I aim to post twice a day, providing you with tips, tricks, motivation, workouts, diet plans and so much more to help you lose weight. Not to mention that I may host a few book giveaways every now and then. In a community, your chance of reaching your goals is much stronger and you may make many new friends in the process!

So, if you are looking for that extra help, please join my Free Facebook Group: https://www.facebook.com/groups/workoutforweightloss

# Chapter 1 – Where do You Stand?

Are you excited to cut the extra pounds to drop the love handles or flatten the round stomach? Firstly, it is a good idea that you know where you stand when it comes to fitness.

It's good to know where you stand so you can plan your next steps towards your final goal. If you are in a position where you haven't exercised in months for whatever reason it may be, or you are obese, then I feel as if the first book of this series "Circuit Training for Beginners" would be more beneficial to you as it will provide you with all the basics and will put you in a great position to start your weight loss journey.

If you are just an average person who exercises every now and then and is looking to lose weight, this book is a good match for you. Most people find themself in your situation, they're carrying a bit of fat, they're not a big fan of exercising, they enjoy occasional snacks and want to do as little as possible to lose it due to their busy lifestyle.

Unfortunately, there's no magic when it comes to losing weight. This book focuses on the simple science of nutrition and exercise to help slim you down to provide you with mental and physical benefits. As you most likely have some previous experience with exercise and nutrition, you will feel comfortable understanding the information in this book. Even if you don't know what circuit training is, those sport sessions you had back at school would have given you all the experience you need to follow this book and get into great shape.

There are many reasons to why you may be reading this book, it may be because you want to start exercising at home, you are looking for quick exercises as you are busy, you don't know how to lose weight, you are bored of running and the list could keep going. What matters is that you are here to lose weight and I will help you do that efficiently.

After reading this opening chapter, I hope you know where you stand, and you are now ready to get into a brilliant workout routine to lose weight. The weight loss won't be instant because that's unrealistic, but you should notice your energy levels rising over time, your body feeling lighter after each exercise and I am sure you will be proud of yourself throughout your weight loss journey. You are going to make a great change to your health and begin to look great in a mirror!

To those of you who read the first book, thank you, I appreciate your decision to stick with me as your virtual trainer and I am also proud of you for sticking with it. This book will carry on from where I left off with the prequel. Although don't worry if this is the only book you want to read from the series because it can be read and understood without references from the other two books. Time to get back to basics...

**Back to Basics**

I am not going to cover the entire book "Circuit Training for Beginners" in this recap as that wouldn't provide any new content for you, instead I will briefly go over some basics to remind you of the foundations. Having strong foundations are important with training so then I can get advanced and into detail throughout this book.

**Circuit Training**

Circuit Training is the training method that this series is centered around. This method of training can be used in so many ways to train many things, but for this instance I am writing this book to help the reader use circuit training in their routine to help them lose weight. You may get sick of seeing the words "Circuit Training", but you will certainly love to complete a circuit after reading this book.

Circuit Training is a workout technique involving a combination of exercises performed in rotation with minimal rest. Each circuit should have 6 or more exercises included and there are countless exercises that you can include in these circuits.

I believe circuit training to be the best training method for you to train because:

Circuit Training is Time-Efficient: The circuits in this book are very quick to set up and takes around 30 minutes to complete.

Circuit Training is Practical: A circuit can be set up anywhere at any time, the circuits in this book require no equipment. So, as we are currently in lockdown you can find a bit of open space at home and get a real good sweat on.

Circuit Training has Variety: You can fit absolutely any exercise into a circuit so that it allows you to train how you like, for example if you are looking to become stronger you can easily set up exercises that will work certain muscles. You can also train with the exercises in different order, train in different areas and so on to provide variety to prevent boredom.

Circuit Training is Easily Modified: Below lies a list of the variables that anyone can change and apply to the circuit, changing a certain variable will provide a different outcome for the Athlete. (The Brackets are Examples)

- Number of exercises in the circuit. (6-12)
- The number of sets (How many times you complete the entire circuit)
- The time spent doing each exercise. (30 seconds)
- The time spent resting between each station. (30 seconds)
- How long to rest after a set. (Around 3 minutes)
- Intensity (measure your heart rate to determine the intensity)
- What exercises to include. (Pushups)
- How many days a week you train (4)

Circuit Training is for Anyone – Can be done if you are any shape and size because it can be modified to suit you. I take considerate of any difficulties people may face like joint problems and I make circuits including exercises that don't require the Athlete to bend their joints.

Circuit Training is Fun – This method of training is much different to going on a run. It has a great range of exercises that will get you moving. You can always complete a circuit with another person, you can complete a circuit with music on or anything you like to make it enjoyable for you. If training is enjoyable then you are motivated.

## Diet

Diet is another key part of these books, I spend a long time researching diet for my books as there are so many different types of diet for example the Keto diet has recently become popular. However, I like to ignore all this stuff and write down the complete basics because they don't come with certain side-effects and work a treat.

In the previous book I provided basic dieting advice along with a week's diet plan and lots of recommended meals that you can include in your day. This book goes further into the reasons for a healthy diet with information on how diet affects your body and brain.

## More Than Just an Exercise Book

If you have read the last book then you know it's more than just listing 10 exercises and calling it a circuit. It went deeper and discussed the problems that come with a lack of exercise and obesity, why everyone should have an exercise routine. There is a huge correlation between the state of the body and mind.

In this book I continue to dive deeper into the correlation between the body and mind, by this I mean that there is factual information on why treating your body right is vital for keeping happy. Motivation, the food and drink we consume, our lifestyle, the things you can do outside of training to boost your gains, how you exercise and most importantly your mindset.

## Training Zones

Intensity and Heart Rate is important to know from the last book. These books require you to work at a required intensity to reach goals, meaning you will have to learn how to measure intensity. Intensity is a measurement of how hard you work while exercising, this can be measured at the rate which your heart is beating per minute. The higher your heart rate the higher the intensity of your workout is. Below are the

Training Zones that I refer to in the descriptions of the circuits, so it is important that you take in this information.

**Very Light** – 50-60% of max heart rate. This is for when you slowly raise your heart rate during a warmup or for people recovering from injury. Walking is an exercise in this range.

**Light** – 60-70% of max heart rate. This is also known as the fat burning zone. You should be able to exercise at this level for a long time, this zone will help you burn fat and improve muscular endurance. A good warmup would take place in this zone.

**Moderate** – 70-80% of max heart rate. This zone is great form improving blood circulation around your heart and skeletal muscles, you will get a bit of a sweat from this zone. Training in this zone is also good for burning fat.

**Hard** – 80-90% of max heart rate. You will breathe harder and work aerobically. At this intensity you will improve your speed endurance and get used to having lactic acid in your blood. I do not recommend working in his zone for a long period as this may result in injury.

**Maximum** – 90-100% of max heart rate. Your body will be working at maximum capacity, you can only train in this zone for short periods of time as lactic acid builds up quickly in blood and can cause cramp or injury. If you are less experienced with training then definitely stay away from this zone.

These training zones are based on your heart rate, this is the best way to measure intensity because your heart works at a different rate to other people in certain circumstances. For the circumstance of exercise, the more active/fit the athlete is then the harder they must work to get their heart rate into the hard training zone than someone who rarely exercises. This is because the athlete's body would have adapted to their lifestyle of regular exercise meaning your heart won't be beating as much than somebody with less athletic traits.

You will need to be able to measure your max heart rate (HR) in order to find out what heart rates you should be working between for certain circuits. You can discover what your maximum heart rate is by subtracting your age from 220. For example, if you are 20 years old then you would have a max heart rate of 200bpm (200-20=200).

You will use your max heart rate to work out what heart rate you should be working between. I will use the light training zone as an example here. To find the lower percentage of the training zone (60% for light zone) you will have to do divide your max heart rate by 100 and times that new number by 60 (200 / 100 = 2 X 60 = 120 bpm), next you will do the same but times that number by 70 instead of 60 to find the higher percentage of the training zone (200/ 100 = 2 X 70 = 140bpm). If you are 20 years old and looking to work in the light training zone, then you will be lucky enough to have to work in between the nice round numbers 120bpm and 140bpm.

**Example Circuit**

Now that I have quickly gone through the basics, here is how I lay out all the circuits involved in this book. I start with listing a few instructions, the first one will be how many sets to complete – this is the number of times you should complete the circuit. Secondly, I state how long to rest in between each exercise, for most circuits it is 30 seconds – please note that this not the same as the rest period between sets. The rest between sets is longer because you need to recover to get into another circuit, I may also word this as rest for 3 minutes after completing the first set. I then set you a target of what heart rate/training zone you should work at – the previous sub-chapter explains this. I finally state the time it takes to complete the warmup, circuit and cooldown.

Complete 2 sets, rest for 30 seconds between each exercise with a 3-minute rest between each set. Train at the Light Training Zone (Around 60% of Max HR). This circuit takes roughly 20 minutes to complete including the warmup and cooldown.

Warmup 2

7. Pushups – 30 seconds

8. Marching on the spot – 30 seconds

9. Calf Raise – 30 seconds

10. Half Squats – 30 seconds

11. Knees to Chest – 30 seconds

12. Jog on the spot – 30 seconds

Cooldown 2


At the top and bottom of the circuit I include the phrase "Warmup 2" and "Cooldown 2", to avoid confusion – that is there because it should remind the reader to warmup before the circuit and cooldown after the circuit. "Warmup 2" is the name of a warmup that is provided in this book, you will need to be familiar with the warmups and cool down I provide in this book as you will be doing them before and after every circuit.

## Equipment

You may look at this subchapter and think "Oh for god's sake, I have just bought another book which says it doesn't require me to buy any equipment but there is a whole sub-chapter dedicated to it.". Hold your horses because I can say with my chest that equipment is **not needed** for any of the circuits – which means you can exercise for free. I think that body weight exercises are the best for losing weight – don't get me wrong equipment can help with losing weight. Also note that you may already have some of the optional equipment that I list.

If you already go to a gym and you are focusing on just weight loss, then you could potentially save yourself money by cancelling your membership and using my book to train at home. At the end of the day, I want all the readers to be satisfied so if I can help you save money along your weight loss journey then I am satisfied myself. If you also have some parts of equipment laying around at home then great, get your money's worth and try to use them in certain exercises – for example you can hold hand weights during burpees for the extra challenge.

Below is a list of a few bits of equipment with an explanation to why you may find them helpful. Please note that I am not telling you to spend money on these products, I am giving an unbiased opinion that will hopefully help you decide whether to get them or not.

**Fitness Mat** – This is just a small soft matt that you can place on the floor to perform your exercises on. You will certainly sweat during these circuits, if you don't want to get your floor sweaty then the fitness matt will soak up the sweat. Also consider how comfortable you would feel exercising on the floor, not every exercise provided is a standing exercise so a matt would be great for providing comfort for your body when on the ground.

**Smart Watch** – There are many different brands of smart watches that all have different capabilities, but I ideally suggest you get a watch that tracks your heart rate. Smart Watches are pricey, and I totally understand if you are against purchasing one. However, it is important that you know what heart rate you are working at so that you don't underwork or overwork. You can calculate your heart rate by measuring your pulse over 15 seconds and times that number by 4 – however I think that will be very hard to do while completing exercises. Instead, you can just simply look at your watch and decide whether you are working at the correct HR or not. It is also beneficial to keep track of the time while exercising so you know when to rest.

**Clothing** – It's a good idea to have the correct attire for when working out. Some brands of clothing are more expensive than others for the reason of the quality, however I am not going to urge you to get a certain brand. A top, shorts/leggings and trainers are all you need to throw on a get a good workout in. Wearing the correct attire can actually motivate you to exercise and most importantly they can soak up sweat better than any other clothing available, at the end of the day you don't really want to try exercise in jeans and a nice top.

**Foam Roller** – This piece of equipment is great for SMR which is later explained, to keep it short SMR is a form of recovery. The foam rollers are used on parts of your body where your muscles may feel tight and allow the tension to be released from muscles. Foam rollers are also helpful for improving flexibility. I suggest having one laying around for when you do feel sore after a workout but it's up to you.

The Circuit Training Weight Loss Bundle that I linked at the start of this book contains all of the links to find all the equipment above for a reasonable price. Sorry to be repetitive, but I want to mention again they are only optional!

# Chapter 2 – Why Mental Strength > Physical Strength

Life is not exactly easy for most people. Mental disorders like Anxiety and Depression are getting more common each day, the most common cause of certain mental disorders is a buildup of stress or a traumatic experience. You can get stressed from many daily activities, it is normal of course but it is how you deal with it what will affect your mental state. It is no-good holding it all in because that makes matters worse. Instead, you have to distract your mind from the stress of life through other activities and let it out in a controlled way. These activities can be anything you enjoy but as you are probably able to tell, I am going to let you know why regular exercise is the best way to relieve stress which allows you to have a positive mental wellbeing. This will give you an insight into the mental side of training and how exercise is more than just getting sweaty.

**The Reason you are Reading**

Let's be real here, there is a reason why you are reading and that will be mainly to lose weight. That's great that you can recognize the problem and you have purchased this book to find a solution. But the problem of being overweight can go much deeper than just looking fat, this subchapter goes into detail why an unhealthy lifestyle doesn't do anybody any favors.

An unhealthy lifestyle is a way of life that includes partaking in activities that are detrimental to your physical and mental well-being. The common activities that may contribute towards your unhealthy lifestyle are things such as: Constant snacking, eating too much, drinking too much, spending too long in front of TV, smoking, not exercising and not maintaining a balanced diet.

It may be slightly harsh of me to guess problems of people who I have never even seen before, but for those who live the unhealthy lifestyle I am going to start with assuming you are overweight or you are not happy with your body. I was once in that situation and from personal experience I can say that it wasn't the happiest stage of my life, I was constantly demotivated, I lacked energy and I wasn't proud to look in the mirror. I know many other people find themselves in that position and it does get to you.

The problem of being overweight is more than just looking fat. There are a huge range of potential health and mental issues. Below is a list of the health-related issues that will hopefully wake you up:

- Type 2 Diabetes
- High Blood Pressure
- Heart Disease and Strokes
- Cancer
- Kidney Problems

They are just a few of the health issues. Although it is not guaranteed that you will suffer from these health issues if you are overweight you still have a higher chance of getting diagnosed with those issues than people who live a healthy lifestyle. Body Mass Index is a good indicator of how overweight you are and if you have a higher chance of being exposed to the health issues. The higher your BMI the greater the chance, a BMI between 25 and 29.9 is healthy so anything above 30 needs to be worked on.

The health issues can range to a life of restrictions (Type 2 Diabetes – having to cut down on what you can eat), or end in death (Heart Disease, Stroke or Cancer). At the end of the day, you want to avoid these issues, so have a look at your unhealthy lifestyle and consider whether it increases or decreases the chances.

It is not just physical issues, here are a few mental issues that being overweight has a potential link of causing:

- Depression
- Anxiety
- Lack of Confidence
- Demotivation

Of course, you are not guaranteed to become diagnosed with depression or anxiety for being overweight, but the lifestyle of someone who is overweight is more likely to make the person lack confidence and motivation which can lead to any mental issues. I was once demotivated due to my weight and not having enough energy all day long, it made me realize that I had to change my lifestyle to enjoy my days living on the earth. As we all know, our days on earth are limited so it is best we make the most out of them.

Other problems with being overweight consist of what you are putting into your body. You will lack energy and not allow your body to perform to the best of its ability. Our brains function best when we eat a balanced and nutritional diet, the good foods that contain fatty acids, antioxidants, vitamins and minerals will nourish the brain and protect it from oxidative stress. Processed foods are often low in fiber so that they can be digested quickly, meaning they can cause swings in blood sugar levels. The sudden changes in blood sugar levels can be harmful to the brain and affect mood.

I believe everything I have talked about in this chapter links together, for example if you are unfortunate enough to have high blood pressure then that will force you to restrict what you can eat/drink which may have a negative effect on your mental state. Other problems like Cancer are much more extreme so you could just imagine how you would feel after being diagnosed with cancer.

Even if you are at a healthy weight, I hope this information will persuade you to get stay away from the unhealthy lifestyle. I talked about these problems in a similar way in the first book so look at this as a reminder why you should make the change, or if you didn't know then great!

Because now you are woken up and hopefully motivated to make the change.

Also note, just because you are at a healthy weight doesn't mean you can't live an unhealthy lifestyle. Eventually, the poor habits will catch up to you and it is harder to get from overweight to a healthy weight than maintaining a healthy weight.

**Resolving the Problems**

There are many ways to cope with the problems I have previously listed. Although I listed a wide range of problems, the solution I am about to explain will be able to lower the risk of health issues and reduce the stress to prevent or calm down mental issues. I do not claim to be able to reverse mental illnesses, I simply have information that I am grateful to pass on as it may help people in their own way.

Exercise. Any form of physical activity is proven to relieve stress. Exercise and other forms of physical activity produce endorphins – endorphins are chemicals in the brain that act as natural painkiller – to which allows your mind to rest, improves your ability to sleep, therefore relieving stress. A relief of stress will certainly make you feel better each day and take your mind to a better place.

Not only are you going to feel great after an exercise, but you will also look great. Well, exercising once isn't going to transform your body like a Greek God's/ Goddess'. But a routine where you exercise a few times a week (Over 150 Minutes of Weekly Physical Activity) will certainly make some positive changes to your body over time. Below is a list of benefits that are caused by exercising consistently:

Strengthens Bones and Muscles – Being strong is useful for Men and Women. There are countless reasons why it is good to be strong, improves your self-defense in unexpected circumstances, may help you for your job, makes you look more attractive and so on...

Helps to keep your thinking, learning and judgement skills sharp – Exercise allows your body to release proteins and other chemicals to improve the function and structure of your brain.

Reduces risk of some cancers, reduces risk of heart disease and increases life expectancy – these are obviously great reasons to exercise as you will enjoy life for longer.

Improves your sexual health – Always an embarrassing subject for some but will reduce chance of erectile disfunctions for men and increase sexual arousal for both genders.

Diet is also another factor that can make a positive contribution to your health mentally and physically, however that is the content of another chapter that will include a template on how to structure your day of eating.

Overall, the way to resolve the problems that come with an unhealthy lifestyle is to reverse the components that make up an unhealthy lifestyle. The lifestyle is mainly made up of watching **too much** TV or eating **too much** food, this should make you realize that a balance is important to achieve a healthy lifestyle.

## What is Your Goal?

If you are reading this book, I hope that you have a goal that includes losing weight. You may want to lose weight to appear slimmer or to look ripped after bulking. But I want your goal to be more than just lose weight. I want it to be specific towards you. Something like losing 5 pounds in 3 weeks, or to get to a flat stomach. I am not here to judge you for your goal, just as long as it is achievable and suits you.

Setting a goal(s) is important because that will allow you to work towards something and brings you motivation. If you don't know how much weight you want to lose or what you want your body to look like, then you won't be as bothered with working out.

If you have a goal like "I want to be happy", then you have to think what factors will make you happy. I too, have a goal to be happy and I believe I can achieve that by maintain a balance of work, relaxation, hobbies and exercise.

It is up to you to set your goals, set a short-term, a medium-term and long-term goal. This way you will never not have anything to work towards to and you can see if you are on track towards your long-term goal. The short-term goal should be set for a few weeks away (6 weeks I suggest), a medium term goal can be from 3-6 months away and long term can be a year away. Write down these goals so you can refer to it.

If you are struggling to set these goals, then continue to read this book and check out my six-week plan. Hopefully, that will inspire you on how to set your goals. I am not willing to set a general goal for all my readers as everyone is different when it comes to weight, height, gender, time available for exercise.

## The Mindset to Hit Goals

I believe mindset is everything when it comes to achieving anything in life. The people who have everything they dreamed about as a kid had to make them sacrifices to get to that position in life later. That's why in the previous sub-chapter I asked you to write down your goal. Writing down your goal is a good way to visualize the route you will take towards reaching your goal. Your path to your goal will be much simpler once laid out, making it much more enjoyable on your weight loss journey. Getting back to making sacrifices, this word often sounds extreme but believe me sacrifices need to be made to reach goals. Even if your sacrifice is to stop drinking on weekends or however simple it may be, you will thank yourself for it later on. So try to think about what sacrifices you can make to reach your goal, and stick to them!

It is up to you to meet these goals. This book will provide you with all the information you need to meet these goals, there is just one last thing – motivation. Motivation is the last piece to the puzzle to reach your goals, because if you know what to do and how do it, but you're not actually doing it then you will not reach your goals - it is as simple as that.

Another key factor of the correct mind set is to think long term. By thinking long-term I mean you should put off the idea of having a quick unhealthy snack or skipping a circuit session because it won't let you progress towards your goals. Develop a mental block that stops you cheating your routine.

## Motivation

I am sure many of you that live the unhealthy lifestyle know the consequences that come with it. You know you should do something about it you still go about your days as normal, or you tried to start a healthy lifestyle but you gave up because it was too challenging. Motivation is a massive factor for many athletes and people in general. Motivation is what stops you giving up when it gets too tough and makes you feel good about yourself. Motivation is that voice in your head that pushes you harder and harder until you reach your goals, there are many ways to become motivated which you can discover below.

**Plan out what you are going to do** – When most people write down a new plan or idea, they often get excited for it. This excitement acts as motivation as it makes you want to exercise, so plan out a new fitness routine to follow. Please read the rest of this book before doing so as it may impact how you write it out.

**Get into Routine** – Now this is the best advice I could offer anyone. If you plan out how you are going to train and you stick to it every week then eventually you will get used to it, you won't even realize it because it will seem so natural for you once you are carrying out the same training each week. A routine has a number of benefits like:

**Improved Sleep** – This will improve your sharpness, performance and energy level throughout the day. Look for at least 8 hours every night, sleep is also vital for rest and recovery.

**Take regular breaks** – This can link to the fitness plan/routine you create. Regular breaks will allow your body and mind to rest and prepare for your next exercise. This creates a balance in your routine – over-working will create stress in your body and mind and potentially cause injury. Injury is a bummer as it won't allow you to exercise for a while, may demotivate you which will cancel out your progress towards your fitness goals.

**Have the workout attire** – Wearing sporting clothing while exercising is a great motivational factor many people look past. You will be working out at home which may feel weird to many people because home is where you usually relax, wearing that relaxing clothing like pajamas or a dressing gown will certainly not make you want to exercise, just instead sit in front of the TV. That's why if you throw on shorts and a top you will instantly feel like you must exercise, your mind will think like this because of how you are dressed. Plus, who would want to get sweaty pajamas anyway?

**Set Realistic Goals** – I know I have talked about this before, but it really is important that you set a short-term, medium-term and long-term goal. This will allow you to always have something to work towards.

**Celebrate when you reach your goals** – Just a follow up from the previous point. Celebrating your goals will make you proud of what you have done and boost your morale. You can choose how you celebrate your goals, maybe a little party or just something fun so that it makes you want to achieve more of your goals so you can have more celebrations. Remember that you should never have no goals, because if you celebrate your final goal you will now not have anything to work towards and it may have a poor effect on you mentally. You have to enjoy life, its only right.

**Track your progress** – Keep on top of your gains towards your goals, because if you don't know how much weight you have lost then how do you know if you are on track to hit your targets. It is motivating to see what you have achieved each week meaning it will encourage you to keep going.

**Enjoy it** – If you enjoy something then you won't complain about doing it right? That's why I try to make the circuits fun so that you won't complain about putting in the hard work. Variety can make it fun because it means you won't get bored of doing the same thing week in week out.

## Achieve that Balance

Hopefully from reading the previous sub-chapter you are now motivated or at least know what will keep you motivated but like with most things in life you should never get over-motivated. There is a difference between being motivated and over-motivated.

When somebody is over-motivated they will likely to be more energetic than usual, their mind will constantly be racing, more intense thoughts about how training went and overall more intense feelings. These intense emotions can bring the worst out of someone.

Being over-motivated can lead to the person over-exercising. Exercising too often can come with consequences like:

- Needing a longer recovery time – could be a potential set back.
- Constantly feeling tired – exercise requires lots of energy.
- Sore muscles/ Heavy Limbs – Will make exercise less enjoyable and a higher risk of getting injured.

- Becoming ill more frequently – just generally not nice.
- A higher chance of injury – this is obvious and can be a major setback. Once you are injured you need to rest and recover until you are fit again and in this time period you will be reversing your progress towards your goals.

In order to have a balance you will have to consider how you can balance out all of your daily activities. For example, if you have 3 hours spare each day then you can break it up into 30 mins of exercising, spending an hour with family, spending an hour on hobbies like gaming and 30 mins reading. Although that is an example it balances out your day so that you feel you haven't given anything too much attention but at the same time you haven't forgotten to do anything.

From this sub-chapter I want you to take away that you shouldn't be doing too much or too little. Finding the right balance is like finding the biting point of the clutch. Doing too much everyday will burn you out and doing too little won't let you progress. Don't only have this mindset for training, but for everything in life. I can personally say that a balanced life brings happiness, yet again I don't want to claim to be able to make anyone happy but at the same time it will improve your mental health.

## Extra Mental Health Advice

I understand that not everyone will want to make a complete change to their lifestyle, so this sub-chapter only contains suggestive information. But the information provided is to help you focus on self-progression and to keep that positive attitude. Having a positive mindset will help you tackle most challenges you face in life efficiently, this book offers more than just training advice because I value my audience.

Spend less time on social media – Today the likes of Instagram, Facebook and Snapchat are all becoming linked to diagnosis of mental issues. Instagram is the worst I believe as all you see on there are pictures of people when they are at their happiest or an achievement of some sort, as humans we compare ourselves to that "Happy" picture of a person and automatically think how poor are lives are – I find myself comparing my living situation to others which isn't great. That is the general assumption is made but it isn't true because that is a photo which does not describe their lifestyle, it only captures a few seconds of their lives which may not be as glamourous as thought.

Have something to look forward to – I have found this difficult to do so in 2020 as pretty much everything enjoyable got cancelled, but this book isn't about me it's about you. Having something to look forward to makes your future look bright and will bring you a feeling of excitement, so try to make plans with friends or family for something that you will all enjoy. This is also another motivation tip but is mainly good for your mental health.

Clear your mind – When you get into a stressful position then you need to stop what you are doing that is causing the stress, whether the cause is work that needs to be done or you are mid-argument with somebody then it is a good idea to stop. Stop and go on a walk, listen to music or anything to take your mind off the stress because you can always come back to finish the work or resolve the argument.

**Extra Benefits Caused by Exercising**

What I don't want to happen is for someone to read this book and still think that exercise is not worth it. Surely these facts below will persuade and motivate you to start exercising and to stop eating junk.

It is medically proven that people who perform regular exercise have:

- up to a 35% lower risk of coronary heart disease and stroke.
- up to a 50% lower risk of type 2 diabetes.
- up to a 30% lower risk of depression.
- up to a 30% lower risk of dementia.
- up to a 83% lower risk of osteoporosis.

Performing regular exercise boosts the ability of your brain. To go into detail, many chemicals are released from the brain during exercise which allow you to become more creative and just be sharp all the time. Being sharp and creative is a huge benefit because it will help you learn, perform at your job well, ignore distractions and achieve greatness.

Other benefits of exercise have already been emphasized throughout this chapter. The only negative I can think of is saying no to a quick chocolate bar, although I can still enjoy a snack every now and then because balance is important remember? In all seriousness the benefits certainly outweigh the negatives by a country mile.

**Do You Want It?**

Think about that question, do you want it? It is easier to say that you are going to do something than actually do it. Think about everything that I have talked about in this chapter and how they link. Does the problem you have make you think in a negative way? Will a change to your lifestyle improve your mental and physical state and solve your problem? Are you motivated enough to stick to your new routine/lifestyle?

These questions are just some that you should think about to motivate you. You have to realize that in order to reach your goals and feel proud doing so, you have to put in that hard work – there aren't any shortcuts. There will be points when you are exercising where you feel that you cannot finish and you want to give up, there will be points where you struggle to get out of bed to train or follow a diet. I promise you that if ignore your negative self-consciousness by getting up and following your routine then you will get through it and feel great doing it!

I hope that you can take something valuable from this chapter and allow it to motivate you to make a change to your lifestyle if it is needed. I once experienced a dark time of my life, I believe that everything I have talked about had helped me mentally. I am not here to compare my bad experience with other peoples as I know some people have been through worse than me. Overall, this chapter is likely to bring value to many people who may not be so well off mentally.

# Chapter 3 – How to Eat for Weight Loss

Most people know that diet is a factor that goes hand in hand with exercise and should be looked at properly. If you think that's a myth, then just look at the top athletes that pay out many thousands on the top nutritionists and dieticians to make sure they perform well in training and in the games. Most people know what they have to sacrifice in terms of food and drink however cannot bring themselves to do it. This chapter will run through the ins and outs of diet, facts on what your body requires every day, examples of food and drink to consume and avoid plus much more. I hope for this information to persuade people to reconsider their diet options.

**Nutrients = Energy**

Below is a detailed evaluation of the six essential nutrients (and fiber) which will help you understand what the body needs to function at its best, while also proving that a balanced diet allows you to get everything you need to maintain high energy levels and train to the best of your ability to lose weight.

**Water** – Consume a minimum of 2.5L per day. Water is extremely important for our body and brain, after all we couldn't live a few days without it. Water carries nutrients to all cells in our body and oxygen to the brain, it allows the body to absorb minerals, vitamins, amino acids, glucose and more, water flushes out waste and toxins, water regulates body temperature and finally water keeps us hydrated. Consume between 2.5L of water to 3.5L everyday to help the body and brain function to the best of its ability. Did you know the body cannot store water? The body uses water so efficient that every drop consumed is used for breathing, sweating and released through urine.

**Protein** – 30% of your daily diet should consist of foods/supplements that are high in protein. Your body needs around 0.75g of protein per kilo of your body weight, using myself as an example 80 x 0.75 = 60 grams of protein every day. If you are looking to build muscle, then you will need at least double that. Eggs, lean meats, poultry, salmon, beans, cheese, and natural peanut butter are all foods that are high in protein, with there being many more foods out there with similar protein properties. I also find protein shakes to be incredible protein providers.

Protein is important because it builds and repairs tissues, helps fight infection and is another source of energy. A lack of protein will leave you weak and tired all the time which will demotivate you and nobody wants that!

**Carbohydrates** – 40% of your daily diet intake should consist of carbs. Normally, your day of eating would consist of 45% to 65% of carbs – however as you are trying to lose weight, eating too many carbs won't allow that.

Carbohydrates are the body's main source of energy. There are good and bad carbs. The good carbs take longer to be broken down by the body and used for energy meaning that you have higher energy levels for a longer period, good carbs can be found in Quinoa, Oats, Sweet potatoes, fruit, chickpeas and pasta. Most good carbs are high in fiber.

Bad carbs on the other hand are foods that contain refined carbohydrates such as white flour or sugar, these will give you a short burst of energy, but your energy levels will drop after the buzz is over which isn't great for maintaining high energy levels. You will find refined carbs in chocolate bars, sweets, cakes, cereals and so on – these kinds of foods would be considered junk anyway, although they may be a tasty treat every now and then to enjoy!

**Fats** – 30% of your daily diet should consist of foods high in fat. Many people think that cutting out fats from their diet is the solution to lose weight, I mean it will work but your body will struggle to produce enough energy. There are 4 types of fats: Saturated fats, Trans-fats, Monounsaturated fats and Polyunsaturated fats.

Saturated fats are very bad for you in high quantities because they are high in cholesterol meaning that if you consume too much saturated fat then LDL (bad) cholesterol in your blood will increase, a continuous high LDL cholesterol increases the chance of stroke and heart disease. Most foods contain saturated fat, you should aim to have 6% of your total daily calories taken up by saturated fats, it is still of course important that you have a small amount of saturated fat in your diet.

There are two types of trans-fats, naturally occurring and artificial trans-fats. The naturally-occurring trans-fats are produced in the gut of some animals meaning it can be found in some meat or milk products, while artificial trans-fats are mainly produced in a factory cheaply by adding hydrogen to liquid vegetable oils. Junk food like doughnuts, frozen pizza, cookies and more are all high in trans-fats. Trans-fats are also bad for you because they raise your LDL (bad) cholesterol and lower HDL (good) cholesterol which increases risk of developing stroke, type 2 diabetes and heart disease.

Monounsaturated fats are considered "good fats" and are mainly found in plant-based liquid oils. These types of fats will reduce you LDL cholesterol when consumed meaning it can reduce the chance of stroke/heart disease. The majority of the fats you eat (So 30% of your daily calorie intake) should be made up of monounsaturated or polyunsaturated fats.

Polyunsaturated fats are another great fat source which can be found in plant-based oils, nuts, seeds and tofu. Similar to monounsaturated fats they lower bad cholesterol levels in your blood. They also provide essential fats that your body needs but can't produce – omega-3 and omega-6 fatty acids.

Eating the correct fat type will certainly help you control your weight, but it most importantly provides your body with the right energy so that it can function to the best of its ability.

**Minerals and Vitamins** – Minerals are a chemical element that contribute towards the body performing well. While Vitamins are an organic compound that also contribute towards the wellness of the body which the human body cannot produce enough of. That means we need to gain minerals and vitamins from out diet to help our body grow, develop and stay healthy. Each mineral and vitamins play a different role to keeping the body healthy and working well, as there are over 20 essential minerals and 13 vitamins I decided to not list all of them with a benefit because that's quite frankly boring.

Some of the main benefits of minerals and vitamins include: strengthening bones, healing wounds and strengthening immune system. They perform well over a hundred roles in the body. An unbalanced diet makes it likely for you to be slightly deficient with some minerals and vitamins but if you follow a healthy/balanced diet then you have nothing to worry about. The essential minerals have a large presence in meat, cereals, fish, dairy products, fruit, vegetables and nuts, as well as being in many other foods. Vitamins have a large presence in leafy green vegetables, plant-based oils, nuts and seeds, meat and dairy products.

From the list above, it is apparent that vitamins and minerals are in most daily foods.

Although, that still allows people to be deficient in a certain mineral or vitamin. As each vitamin or mineral serves a slightly different role to keep the body healthy, a deficiency for each mineral or vitamin will come with different symptom. The most common deficiencies with their problem are in a list below.

- Iron Deficiency (Mineral) – Causes anemia, fatigue, weak immune system and impaired brain function.

- Vitamin D Deficiency (Vitamin) – Muscle weakness, bone loss and increased risk of fractures.

- Magnesium Deficiency (Mineral) – irregular heartbeat, muscle cramps, migraines and fatigue.

- Vitamin A Deficiency (Vitamin) – Causes eye damage, suppresses immune function and may lead to blindness.

I hope that's enough to encourage you to get your vitamins in. There are of course less intense symptoms for those who are only slightly deficient, but they could do with a bit more – you may find yourself to be in this category. Things like dry skin, brittle hair and feeling sleepy all the time is the result of not getting enough minerals or vitamins.

It is a good idea that you eat a balanced diet because that will allow you to avoid the problems recently talked about. You can always take mineral and vitamin tablets to make sure that you meet the required amount each day, I provide a link to tablets later. Of course, it requires a balance like most things in life so there are consequences of too much. Symptoms of overdose may include:

- Nausea
- Diarrhea

- Headache
- Fluid Build Up

**Fiber** – This is not an essential nutrient, nevertheless it is still a nutrient and is useful to know about when aiming for weight loss. Fiber is a non-digestible carbohydrate found in foods, it can be split into soluble fiber and Insoluble fiber which to put it simply soluble fiber can dissolve in water and insoluble fiber cannot. Both types of fiber are great for controlling weight because it can soak up water in the intestine which will slow down the rate which nutrients are absorbed and increase the feeling of fullness. A feeling of fullness will discourage you to snack through the day saving you from that extra weight piling up. The recommended amount of fiber that should be consumed daily is from 25 to 30 grams. Foods that are high in fiber include leafy vegetables, berries, citrus fruits, nuts, seeds, wholegrain oats and beans.

From this subchapter I mainly want you to understand what you should and shouldn't be putting into your body as it has a knock-on effect to your physical and mental health. There have been many foods and food groups listed in this chapter that supply your body with these nutrients, which will also be included in the example diet plan, the next paragraph will give examples of what you should avoid which may be in your daily diet right now.

You should be cutting junk food, unhealthy snacks and sugary drinks out of your diet. These kinds of foods have low nutritional value and are usually high in saturated fat or sugar which you know aren't good for you. Foods labelled as junk food are things like Pizza, fried food, grilled food,

French fries, Burgers, fast food and most takeaways. Unhealthy snacks are things like chocolate bars, sweets, sweetened cereal bars, crisps, pastries and biscuits. Finally, you should avoid sugary drinks like Coca-Cola, putting sugar in tea or coffee, milkshakes and although alcoholic drinks aren't typically sugary, they should still be avoided because they contain many calories. I understand it is a complete change to just cut out some of your favorite snacks and treats, in the weeks plan I allow you to have a cheat meal – this acts as motivation and it is also an extreme challenge to cut your favorite foods out of your diet completely. A cheat meal is a meal where you can eat anything you like and make sure you enjoy it.

## Do you have Breakfast?

May sound like a weird question, but do you actually sit down in the morning and eat a nutritional breakfast? I ask this because many people don't, I found this fact shocking that surveys say over half of the UK population skip breakfast every morning as they can't find time for it. A large number of people have the nutritionally incorrect breakfast alongside the large number of people who don't bother. I am here to address this issue and get everyone reading this to have a great breakfast.

If you have an unhealthy breakfast which consists of eating sugary cereal, having a full English or just eating toasted white bread then you are making your body suffer from the moment you wake up. You burn many calories in your sleep and your body needs to be replenished so that it can prepare to maintain the energy for the day. It is ideal for your breakfast to be high in fiber and lower in sugars, while also containing the six essential nutrients. You can find some great breakfast examples in the example diet plan.

## When to Eat

Planning out when you eat is beneficial for many reasons. The main reason is because you will be able to space out your meals, research shows that spacing out your meals into five or six smaller meals will boost your metabolism – while if you continue to have 2 or 3 meals a day then your body will go into "Starvation Mode" before meals - where your body burns your muscles to produce and conserve energy. When you eat one of the 3 meals (which is usually more than the body needs) the body will store the excess energy as fat. Five or six smaller portions where you have a meal once every 3 hours will allow your body to use the energy efficiently. You also need to make sure you eat before and after exercising so that your body has the energy required to complete the exercise.

You also have to be careful when to eat before and after exercise, leaving little time between a meal and exercise will not allow your food to digest properly meaning you will be likely to vomit or you will feel drained as the nutrients/energy would not have set in yet. Alternatively, leaving a long time between eating a meal and exercising is also a bad idea because your energy levels will not be as high as necessary to complete the exercise to a great standard. The ideal time to leave before exercising just after eating a small meal is one to two hours, this means you will easily be able to fit in an exercise between two meals. You should leave 30 minutes after an exercise before you eat. While exercising it is important that you have water with you to keep hydrated because you will be sweating out liquid.

## A Days Dieting Example

In the first book of this series, I listed a week's diets that people could follow or adapt slightly every week to help them progress with weight loss. However, I don't want to repeat myself for those who came from my previous book but at the same time I don't want there to be an insufficient amount of information for the new readers. So below is a days' worth of eating that will show you how often you should be eating, what kind of food you should be eating and will also include some alternative foods for those with certain restrictions.

When losing weight, you want to consume less calories than usual, this doesn't mean for you to starve yourself it's just that you have to be careful which foods you decide to eat. Everyone is different when it comes to the recommended intake of calories they should consume, to work out your recommended calorie intake simply just follow the steps on https://www.calculator.net/calorie-calculator.html .

The day of eating below will allow you to eat 2000 calories while getting a great serving of all the essential nutrients to keep your body energized. This is just an example so please don't feel the need to follow this day every single day as you will get bored of the food choices – there are a few alternatives below the example. But it is a good idea to stick to times provided for each meal as that will keep your metabolism working well, if you did work out your recommended calories then times that figure by 0.8 (80%) to find out how many calories you should be consuming roughly to lose weight. Remember to split the calories across the day so each meal should make up roughly 20% of the recommended weight loss calorie intake.

## Example Day

**Breakfast (6am-9am)**:

Bowl of Porridge with banana slices (300 Calories). 6g fat, 50g carbs – 6g fiber, 11g protein. Take 1 Formula 2 Vitamin & Mineral Tablet

**Mid-Morning Meal (10am-11.30am):**

2 Slices of Whole meal Toast with 2 Tablespoons of Peanut Butter (Around 350 Calories)38g carbs, 9g fat, 7g protein. 1g fiber.

**Lunch (12pm-2pm):**

Chicken breast with 100g basmati rice and half red pepper (Around 400 Calories) 25.22 carbs, 55 grams of protein, 6 grams fat. 1g fiber.

**Midafternoon Meal (2.30pm-4:30pm):**

2 Slices of Beans on Wholemeal Toast (Around 400 Calories) 14g protein, 65 carbs, 6 fat, 12 fiber.

**Dinner (5.30pm-8:30pm):**

Super healthy Salmon Salad (320 Calories) 10g fat, 30g carbs, 2g fiber, 30 protein.

**Snacks (Any time):**

30g of mixed nuts (185 Calories) 16.89g fat, 6.47g carbs, 5g protein, 3g fiber.


**Overview:**

Around 1950 calories – each meal contains roughly 350 to 400 calories to keep the day of eating nice and balanced.

Fat consumed 54g – the majority being polyunsaturated.

Carbs consumed 189g.

Protein Consumed 122g

Fiber Consumed 25g. This just about meets the daily requirements, you will feel full throughout the day and your body will be burning fat by doing so.

If you are looking for alternative meals for what I have provided, then have a look at the diet section in the first book "Circuit Training for Beginners" – I don't want to repeat myself. Failing that you can always search the web for healthy small meals, and you will find countless options.

**Spending Money**

Food will always cost you money, unless you grow and cook your own food every single day then you cannot disagree with that statement. Many people end up spending way too much on food which results in having less money for the bills, clothes and other necessities.

First of all, you should have a look at how much money you spend in a day on food, this may be vegetables, sweets, coffee, takeaways and so on. Then compare it to my days diet plan expenses and you may see that my weeks plan costs less money which means if you follow that or a similar plan then you as well will effectively save money – if you compare the two and notice yours is actually cheaper, fair play, but it also makes me consider if you are eating enough.

A takeaway here and there, with a couple dollars or pounds on unhealthy snacks each day will certainly leave you spending more than you need. It is likely that you will save money when you start eating healthier, you can put that money aside and save up for holidays or days out and you will be glad looking back at your decisions.

I hope that you got what you need from this chapter, I am always looking to improve diet sections of these books and avoid repetition. Just remember, cutting out junk food benefits your body and bank balance.

# Chapter 4 – How to Correctly Prepare for Circuits

Now you have got to the exercise part of the book, finally! This chapter focuses on how you can prepare for circuits so that you complete them to the best of your ability to maximize how quickly you can lose weight.

**Warmups**

A warmup is vital to complete before any form of exercise, that's why I include the warmup with every circuit to remind you to complete it beforehand. Warmups can be varied in any way, as long as it contains stretches for the muscles that are going to be worked and light activities (Heart Raisers), then it is a good warmup. Below are two warmups labeled "Warmup 2" and "Warmup 3", these warmups are different and will match up with the circuits in chapter 6. If you are wondering where warmup 1 is, that is included in the Beginner book because that links with the more basic circuits.

Warmup 2 (4 Minutes)
- Marching on Spot – 1 minute
- Arm Circles – 30 seconds
- Left Right Floor Taps - 1 minute
- Quad Stretch – 15 seconds each leg
- Cross Body Shoulder Stretch – 15 seconds each arm

Warmup 3 (5 Minutes)
- Light Jog on Spot – 1 minute
- Walking Knee Hugs – 30 seconds
- Sexy Circles – 30 seconds
- Arm Extension Hold – 30 seconds
- Ankle Rolls – 30 seconds

- Lateral Split Squat Stretch – 30 seconds
- High Kick Outs – 30 seconds
- Heel Flicks – 1 minute

**Cooldowns**

Cooldowns take place after the workout and typically take around 5 minutes to complete. Cooldowns allow gradual recovery of heart rate and blood pressure. Cooldowns help you relax after a workout so that your recovery time will improve. A good cool-down includes light activities and seated stretches. Cooldown 2 is the only cooldown required for the circuits in this book, just like the warmups – "Cooldown 1" is considered too basic for these circuits and is found in the beginner book. Although this is done after a workout, this is still preparation because it allows recovery which prepares you for the next circuit.

Cooldown 2 (3 Minutes) – Lower Heart Rate to very light training zone

- Shake off Body – 30 seconds
- Side to Side – 30 seconds
- Forward Fold – 30 seconds
- Open the Gates – 30 seconds
- Cross Body Shoulder Stretch – 30 seconds
- Side Leg Raises – 30 seconds

**Rest and Recovery**

You may think that resting and recovering is not preparing for a circuit as you would rest after a circuit, however, you have to take into consideration that you will be training 4 to 5 days a week meaning rest and recovery will be preparing you for a circuit the next day.

Rest is what allows your body to recover along with many other components I list shortly.

Recovery is important in any training routine as it has a big impact on your weight loss, training performance and most importantly allows you to train effectively. After a workout, such as a circuit, your muscles and tissue will be worn out and slightly damaged – slight damage is normal as certain hormones in your body have the job to repair muscles and tissue. It usually takes from 24 to 48 hours to repair naturally, however it only takes this long for weightlifters as they are purposely damaging their muscles to improve strength. Recovery times are different for everyone, but of course can be improved by the action of consistent exercise overtime.

I suggest that it would take roughly 20 hours to recover from a circuit in this book, although that suggests that you would be able to train everyday – that isn't a great idea because the stress will build up in your muscles and damage them for a much longer period than just 20 hours (Injury). That's why training 5 days a week is important because it allows a couple of days for proper rest and recovery, plus you will get at least 20 hours rest between exercise where the training days are back-to-back.

**How to Speed up Recovery**

Below are tips that will help you prepare for the next circuit. These tips will improve how quickly you recover. You will naturally complete some of these tips like resting and replenishing fluids – make sure you look out for the SMR, personally I think that is the most effective.

**Replenish Fluids** – While exercising you lose lots of fluid due to sweating and your body uses water to transport nutrients and energy to the parts of the body that needs it. So always have a bottle of water around while exercising that you can drink during the rest periods or after the circuit. Staying constantly hydrated will speed up your recovery time.

**Rest** – Your body knows how to recover best, and it can do that while you are relaxed. You know how to rest and relax best, for me I would lay on the sofa with my feet up watching some Netflix. So, make sure you put your feet up after a circuit to allow your body to naturally recover. Sleep is a massive part of rest which is usually looked past as it is natural, you should have a minimum of 8 hours sleep each night and set your bedtime before midnight – it is proven that an earlier bedtime and consistent sleep boosts recovery times.

**Stretch** – Stretching muscles after a circuit allows faster recovery because it allows your blood to flow to your muscles. If you complete the cooldown properly after the circuit then you will be stretching properly and improving your recovery time as well as reducing chance of injury.

**Nutrition** – Although this has been covered heavily, I just want to remind you that the correct diet will allow your body to function to a better standard and of course improve recovery time. Eating after a workout will replenish your body with the energy that you have just used up while exercising.

**Posture** – Many people don't pay attention to posture, nowadays more people have a bad posture due to sitting down for many hours each day or being in an unrestful position. People with desk jobs are more likely to suffer. If you have a bad posture or a posture that could be worked on then: focus on stretching and strengthening upper back muscles (exercise helps), always sit up straight or use posture straightening equipment like a back brace. Having a good posture allows your body to be in a good condition which will naturally improve recovery time as well as bring you many benefits.

**Self-Myofascial Release** – This is a form of tool assisted self-massage that will take stress out of your muscles or joints. A foam roller is most common for SMR to massage your muscles after a workout to help with muscle or joint pain. SMR can clear up restrictions and muscle knots, this means that if you have slight aches, knots or pains then using SMR will increase your recovery time significantly and more importantly will prevent you from training with these restrictions or pains which cause injury.

**Thermoregulation** – Cold water immersion is more commonly used nowadays for recovery after a workout. Cold water immersion is best done by getting into an ice bath or having a cold shower for a few minutes – this will cool you down after a workout (prevents overheating) and will reduce blood flow in your muscles which, makes your muscles recover from exercise quicker. Heat can also help your muscles to relax, either a heat pack or a steamy shower will warm up your muscles to allow relaxation. If you want to combine the two you can try a 10-minute shower in which you have 1-minute warm and 1-minute cold continuously for the 10 minutes. The warm-cold interval shower will restrict blood vessels, flush the body with blood and drive the blood inwards which make your organs work better, which lead to better recovery time.

I am not expecting you to try all these recovery tips, however you should try 2-3 on your rest days or right after an exercise. You may find yourself already doing these which is a bonus. I find posture to be the most important because a good posture brings more benefits than just a quick recovery time.

# Chapter 5 – Behind the Scenes of Health & Fitness

This chapter focuses on the things that will help you reach your goals. Although this entire book is designed to do that, this chapter specifically targets things that can be done outside of the fitness routine to boost results. Not to mention that progressive overload, and injury are covered.

## Progressive Overload

This was explained in detail in the previous book, used in the beginner six-week plan and best know it makes an appearance in the intermediate six-week plan. To put it simply, progressive overload is a method of training that requires the exercises to be made more difficult overtime which allows your body to adapt to the training load, which makes you fitter. Progressive overload is mainly used by weightlifters, they make the exercises harder by increasing the weight of the equipment they use so that muscles have a harder time pushing/pulling the equipment and that will cause the muscles to rip and get stronger. As you readers are not weightlifters or not using equipment then you will not be increasing resistance in your workouts, instead you can gradually increase variables like time spent exercising, days a week spent exercising, your heart rate and decreasing rest period. These variables go hand in hand, for example if you decrease the rest periods then you will technically be increasing your heart rate as your heart will have less rest time to slow down.

**Injury**

I am sure that you all know that Injury is something that you should avoid at all costs. If you think injury is a good thing then let me educate you about the cons of injury: Injury will make you unable to exercise until you have properly recovered. Injury can be very painful at times and can send you to hospital which costs in certain parts of the world. There are many different injuries that you can experience, some may be short term and some long term – the most common ways of getting injured while training include:

- Over exhaustion
- Mistakes (slipping/other people causing injury)
- Not stretching.

The most common injuries are muscle strains, ligament damage and ankle sprain.

Below you will find a list of ways to prevent injury with an explanation to help you understand how the body gets injured while exercising.

**Warming Up** – As mentioned before, a warmup is a short combination of heart raisers and stretches which prepares you for exercise. Warmups prevent injuries because the heart raisers slowly raise your heart rate – this prevents your heart rate suddenly increasing rapidly - which doesn't allow enough blood to be pumped around your body and means that your body doesn't get the energy it needs transferred around the body properly. The stretches in the warmup allow your muscles to have an extended range of motion, meaning you are less likely to strain your muscles to any sudden movements.

**Allow Rest/Don't Overtrain** – I think these two go hand in hand because by overtraining you are not allowing yourself enough rest. I have allocated rest periods between exercises so that you get sufficient rest and allocated longer rest in between sets. The reason why rest is important because your body will not be able to cope with constantly working hard for a prolonged period, when your body reaches exhaustion you will become out of breath and your muscles will feel heavy making it hard to continue exercising. If you continue to train during exhaustion, then you are vulnerable to injury. These breaks allow you to avoid complete exhaustion, however there shouldn't be too many breaks as that wouldn't allow you to get your heart rate in the moderate training zone.

**Use Proper Technique** – If you don't know how to properly complete an exercise then it is always a good idea to look up how to do it to avoid embarrassment and injury. Completing an exercise with incorrect form may cause: balance issues - potentially ending with a fall, muscle strain – using certain muscles more than needed and put extra stress on your tendons and joints.

**Wear Correct Clothing** – By this I mainly mean for you to wear appropriate footwear for the floor you will be exercising on – a hard floor will not be kind for your feet, or a slippery floor will not hold your balance. I am not asking you to replace your floor because that's ridiculous just instead you should consider wearing sporting footwear (which typically are light with good grips) to prevent slips, unbalance and provides comfort for your feet. Also wearing fitness clothing will prevent clothing getting caught which may end up in injury.

Preventing injury is mostly done with common sense, don't try to do something if there's a chance you will get hurt. The circuits in this book will make it hard to get injured as they aren't exactly dangerous or extremely difficult, but it is still possible and will put your fitness journey on hold.

**Exercising Tips and Tricks**

Just like everything in life, there are many "Tips" and "Tricks" that help you reach your goal quicker. For exercising, these tips and tricks allow you to train to the best of your ability which speeds up the rate you make progress towards your goal.

**Take Caffeine Before a Circuit** – I am sure many of you wake up and start the day off with a caffeinated drink, that drink most likely being coffee. However, you should have a caffeinated drink of some sort around 60-90 minutes before an exercise, it takes that long for the blood levels to peak after absorbing the caffeine. Caffeine will help you with your workout because it: effects the nervous system – improving focus and energy, enhances hormones – adrenaline that increases performance, improves the body ability to burn and breakdown fats, endorphins – this improves the feeling of wellness and increases body temperature to burn more calories. Overall caffeine improves your energy levels and allows you to exercise to a better standard. Please don't have too much caffeine as it is dangerous, around 100mg of caffeine 90 minutes before a workout is great!

**Breathing Rate** – How you breathe while exercising is more important as you think, most people don't even think about how they breathe because it is natural (hopefully). The overall rule for exercising is for you to inhale while relaxing and exhaling during exertion, this could mean for pushups that you exhale while you lower your chest to the floor and inhale once you return to that standard pushup position momentarily after pushing up – I understand that every exercise is different and it's not right if I explain how to breathe for every single exercise. I suggest that you inhale at the start of the rep and exhale during the rep for most of the exercises. For the quicker exercises like jumping jacks then you will want to inhale for 2 or 3 reps then exhale for 2 or 3 reps and continue to do this. You should be able to know what exercises you can complete quickly and use this knowledge to alter your breathing rate. It is better for you to take deep inhales and longer exhales because this allows more oxygen to get to your muscles and will less likely put you out of breath. At the moderate intensity it is better to breathe through your nose, but that doesn't mean you have to completely avoid breathing through your mouth.

**How to increase lung capacity** – When exercising the one thing that will cause people to stop is when they are completely out of breath, I am not of course going to force you to carry on during exhaustion because that's cruel and dangerous, however I will provide a breathing exercise that will improve lung capacity, this exercise will also help people that are short of breath. Diaphragmatic Breathing: Lay down and relax your shoulders, place one hand on your belly and the other on your chest, then inhale through your nose for two seconds before breathing out through your pursed lips (breathe out as if you are whistling) while pressing on your abdomen. Repeat that breathing technique a few times and increase the duration of inhales and exhales overtime to increase your lung capacity.

**Listen to Music** – Let's be honest, exercising alone in silence is boring and off-putting if the only thing you can hear is heavy panting from yourself. That's why I suggest that you play some music in the background or through headphones. The music that you play should be enjoyable to listen to and that is completely subjective, personally I like to rap as I find the lyrics motivating, the beat enjoyable which pushes me to get through it all. So, get a playlist of songs that you like listening to that you think will help you through the workout.

## How to Deal With Reaching Goals

I don't know what your exact goals are, I understand you are here to lose weight but I'm not sure how much you want to lose, how long you are setting this goal for and so on. What I can provide though is information on what you should do after you reach your goal(s).

I hope that you have set two or three goals, these goals should cover short-term, medium-term and long-term. There is always a chance that you reach your goals quicker than expected – this is not always a good thing because it can lead to people falling out of routine/ losing motivation and you know how that ends.

So, when you reach a goal quicker than expected and you don't have anything to work towards, you should set a new goal or two straight away. One of these goals should be to maintain your previous goal – an example of this could be: if that your goal was to lose 10kg over 3 months and you completed that quicker than expected then you should maintain the weight you are at for however long is necessary. The idea being is you should always have something to work towards, you may think that maintaining a certain weight doesn't make you have to work for it however it is more common for people to pile on the weight again after they reach a goal which means overall, they have made no progress.

Of course, you can set a harder goal after reaching a goal, but just remember if you keep doing this then you will eventually get to an extremely high fitness level which may become more time consuming and clash with other parts of your life. Also, if you just focus on losing weight and keep setting goals higher and higher eventually you will have no weight to lose and being underweight is not healthy. Like I said previously, achieve that balance and get yourself to a level where you are comfortable and happy with yourself.

# Chapter 6 – The Workouts for Weight Loss

Here is the chapter where I list all the circuits for you to complete at home. The chapter after this includes a six-week plan, you can either follow the six-week plan in the next chapter or take inspiration from the next chapter and take the exercises/circuits to create your own training plan. I'm not bothered how you do it, just as long as you do it.

In this chapter you will find 8 circuits. You will see a pattern to three of the circuits which have the name "Medium Impact Circuit 1", "High Impact Circuit 1" and "High Impact Circuit 2" – all of these "Impact" circuits will be used in the intermediate fitness six-week plan. Those three circuits will be varied with the exercises, for example the circuits will have a mixture of standing exercises, floor-based exercises and each circuit will work most of the muscle groups in the body to provide balance and allow you to burn fat evenly across the body. The HIIT taster circuit also makes a short appearance!

If you don't feel like following the six-week plan, then no worries as you can still use them three circuits plus many more to include in your routine. The additional circuits all have their own specialties, for example the "Floor Circuit" contains many exercises that are completed on the floor for a great body workout. My personal favorite is the "Abs Burnout Circuits (The ABC)", this is a circuit that contains a range of exercises that target the abs and obliques that will also help you lose weight to get a shredded six-pack.

I have included a big range of exercises and their descriptions so hopefully you will not feel the need to search up any more after reading any of the circuit training books. I understand that many people have restrictions which may include joint pain, back pain other reasons, these restrictions will make certain exercises hard to complete as it may be painful or uncomfortable to complete. My advice is to check with a doctor if you can complete the exercises listed in the next chapter, or you can check out the first book of the series which has easier exercises. I suggest those who are held back by these restrictions to not complete the circuits below until you are comfortable with completing a beginner circuit.

## How Often to Exercise

The NHS suggest that all adults that don't suffer from difficulties or conditions should complete a minimum of 150 minutes of moderate activity per week or 75 minutes of vigorous activity per week. These circuits have been designed to be moderate meaning you should complete a minimum of 150 minutes of exercise per week.

It may sound like a lot but trust me it is worth it and once you are in a routine you won't even notice. Exercise 5 days a week by completing a circuit in each of the days you are exercising, use the six-week plan included further on in this book for inspiration. If you train 5 days a week with these circuits which are all around 30 minutes, then you will easily meet the 150-minute requirement. The final circuit provided in this book falls under the category of vigorous activity – so keep that in mind.

**Medium Impact Circuit 1**

You may remember this circuit from "Circuit Training for Beginners", I believe this circuit to be great for those who are transitioning from a beginner to a standard level. This circuit has a great variety of exercises, working most parts of the body with a combination of floor and standing exercises.

Complete 3 sets, rest for 30 seconds between each exercise and rest for 2 minutes after each set. Train at the moderate training zone (Around 70% of Max HR). This circuit will take roughly 30 minutes to complete including the warmup and cooldown.

Warmup 2
1. Jogging on the Spot – 30 seconds
2. Russian Twists – 30 seconds

3. Knee to Chest Taps – 30 seconds

4. Straight Punches – 30 seconds

5. Lying Superman Hold – 30 seconds

6. Tuck Jumps – 30 seconds

7. Crunches – 30 seconds

8. Squats – 30 seconds

Cooldown 2

**High Impact Circuit 1**

Contains a mixture of floor and standing exercises which will certainly allow you to get a sweat on. This is slightly harder than the medium impact circuit as it requires you to work at a higher heart rate.

Complete 2 sets, rest for 30 seconds between exercises and rest for 2 minutes between each set. Train at moderate training zone (Around

75% of Max HR). This circuit including the warmup and cooldown will take 25 to 30 minutes to complete.

Warmup 3

1. Running on the Spot – 30 seconds
2. Knee to Chest Taps – 30 seconds
3. Calf Raise – 30 Seconds
4. Squat Jumps – 30 seconds
5. Left to Right Jabs – 30 seconds
6. Ali Shuffle – 30 seconds
7. Pushups – 30 seconds
8. Squat and Hamstrings – 30 seconds
9. Marching Air Punches – 60 seconds

Cooldown 2

**High Impact Circuit 2**

Complete 2 sets, rest for 30 seconds between exercises and rest for 3 minutes between sets. Train at moderate training zone (Around 75% of Max HR). This circuit including the warmup and cooldown will take 25 to 30 minutes to complete.

Warmup 3

1. Left to Right Jabs – 30 seconds
2. Lateral Split Squats – 30 seconds
3. Left Right Floor Taps – 30 Seconds
4. Forwards and Back Crawl – 30 Seconds
5. Side Lunge – 30 seconds
6. High Knee Twists – 30 seconds
7. Wide Pushups – 30 seconds
8. Heel Flicks – 30 seconds
9. Plank – 60 seconds

**Abs Burnout Circuit**

This circuit is specific to strengthen and tone your abdominals as well as burn belly fat, this circuit will be useful if you have a goal of burning belly fat and in the long run looking for a six-pack. A few other muscles will be worked as well but the primary muscles used are the abdominals and obliques. Make sure that you engage your core for every single exercise included so you get the most work out of your abs.

Complete 2 sets, rest for 30 seconds between each exercise with a 2-minute rest between sets. Train at the moderate training zone (Around 70% of Max HR). It will take roughly 20 minutes to complete this including the warmup and cooldown.

Warmup 2
1. Crunches – 30 seconds
2. Lying Superman Hold – 30 seconds
3. Plank – 30 seconds

4. Ankle Taps – 30 seconds

5. Forwards and Back Crawl – 30 seconds

6. Standing Side Crunch – 30 seconds

7. Russian Twists – 30 seconds

Cooldown 2

**Leg Day Circuit**

This is a circuit that contains exercises that work the legs muscles, these muscles include the Hamstrings, Quadriceps, Calves and Glutes. These exercises will certainly allow you to strengthen your legs which bring many benefits as well as burn body fat.

Complete 3 sets, rest for 30 seconds between each exercise with a 2-minute rest between sets. Train at the moderate training zone

(Around 70% of Max HR). Will take 25 to 30 minutes to complete.

Warmup 3

1. Boxer Squats – 30 seconds
2. Calf Raises – 30 seconds
3. Twist Jumps – 30 seconds
4. Lunges with Twists – 30 seconds
5. Squat Jumps – 30 seconds
6. Lateral Split Squats – 30 seconds

Cooldown 2

**Floor Circuit**

This circuit includes exercises hat can only be performed on the floor. I thought I would make this addition to the book because it provides more variety and why not. The general rule of floor exercise is that they work your upper and lower body, most particularly your core. So, if you are looking for a great whole-body workout, then bobs your uncle. This is also a longer circuit than others so keep that in mind.

Complete 4 sets, rest for 30 seconds between sets and 3 minutes between each set. Train at the moderate training zone (70% of Max HR). Will take from 35 to 40 minutes to complete.

Warmup 2

1. Pushups – 30 seconds
2. Crunches – 30 seconds
3. Forwards and Back Crawl – 30 seconds
4. Wide Pushups – 30 seconds
5. Ankle Taps – 30 seconds
6. Plank – 30 seconds

Cooldown 2

**Pure Cardio Circuit**

The exercises in this circuit are all the kind that will increase your heart rate and make you sweat. You already know the benefits of exercising, but this circuit contains the exercises you need to burn calories to lose weight.

Complete 4 sets, rest for 30 seconds between sets and 3 minutes between each set. Train at the moderate training zone (70% of Max HR). Will take from 35 to 40 minutes to complete.

Warmup 2
1.  Ali Shuffle – 30 seconds
2.  Left Right Floor Taps – 30 seconds
3.  Heel Flicks – 30 seconds
4.  Straight Punches (Quick) – 30 seconds
5.  Forwards and Back Crawl – 30 seconds
6.  Squat Jumps – 30 seconds

Cooldown 2

**HIIT Circuit Taster**

This is a circuit that falls under the HIIT category and will give you a taster to what the circuits from the next book "High Intensity Circuit Training", this will be the toughest circuit included in this book so beware. Remember this circuit counts as vigorous physical activity towards the recommended 75 minutes.

Complete 3 sets, rest for 30 seconds between each exercise with a 3-minute rest between sets. Work at the Hard Training Zone (Around 80% of Max HR). Will take 30 minutes to complete including the warmup and cooldown.

Warmup 3

1. Burpees – 20 seconds

2. Bicycle Crunch – 20 seconds

3. Tuck Ups – 20 seconds

4. Shoulder Pushups – 20 seconds

5. Forward Kick Outs – 20 seconds

6. Open and Close Gates – 20 seconds

Cooldown 2

# Chapter 7 – From Fat to Fit in Six-Weeks

This is starting to become a famous feature in my fitness books. This is where I list a six-week plan that contains circuits that will allow you to get your recommended 150 minutes of exercise each week and give you insights to how a fitness routine should look like.

The second chapter of the book contained the basic information on why a routine is important. Routines can be useful to everyone, for the instance of exercising it works a treat as it is highly motivating. Anyway, this six-week plan can be picked up exactly from where the previous six-week plan was left off. Before you get into the six-week plan you need to make sure you are familiar with the circuits and the exercises included, remember all the training tips that will help you

inside and outside of exercise and most
importantly enjoy it!

Of course, this six-week plan contains
progressive overload because you will get fitter
while training meaning it must get harder over
time. The difficulty of the circuits is presented by
the time allowed to rest, the amount of time
allocated for each exercise and the intensity at
which the exercises are performed at.

**The Six-Week Plan**

**Week 1**

**Monday –**

What to Train: Medium Impact Circuit 1

Progressive Overload Changes: None

**Tuesday –** Rest Day. This goes for every rest day:
Refer to the rest and recovery tips to ensure you
are prepared for the next circuit.

**Wednesday –**

What to Train: Medium Impact Circuit

Progressive Overload Changes: None

**Thursday –** Rest Day

**Friday -**

What to Train: Medium Impact Circuit.

Progressive Overload Changes: Decrease the resting period by 10 seconds. Meaning you spend 20 seconds resting between each exercise.

**Saturday –**

What to Train: High Impact Circuit 1

Progressive Overload Changes: No changes to this circuit, however including this circuit makes it slightly more challenging.

**Sunday –** Rest Day. Great work for this week, now it's time to get onto week 2.


**Week 1 overview:**

The first week should always ease you into the routine so there is nothing too hard here, this week mainly consists of completing the medium impact circuit and completing the high impact circuit once to provide variety and more difficulty. This week contains at least 120 minutes of moderate activity, 30 minutes away from the recommended.

## Week 2

**Monday –**

What to Train: High Impact Circuit 2

Progressive Overload Changes: No changes to this circuit, however it is new to the six-week plan.

**Tuesday –** Rest Day

**Wednesday –**

What to Train: Medium Impact Circuit

Progressive Overload Changes: Increase the duration of the exercise period by 10 seconds, this means that you should spend 40 seconds on each exercise.

**Thursday –** Rest Day

**Friday –**

What to Train: High Impact Circuit 1

Progressive Overload Changes: No new changes –
still getting used to this harder circuit.

**Saturday –**

What to Train: High Impact Circuit 2

Progressive Overload: No new changes.

**Sunday –** Rest Day.


**Week 2 Overview:**

Still easing you into a fitness routine but is
certainly a step up from the previous week. In this
week I include both high impact circuits and
implement progressive overload to the medium
impact circuit so that you spend more time
burning calories. This week includes around 125
minutes of exercise.


**Week 3**

**Monday –**

What to Train: Medium Impact Circuit

Progressive Overload Changes: No new changes, still train 40 seconds per exercise.

**Tuesday –** Rest Day

**Wednesday –**

What to Train: Medium Impact Circuit

Progressive Overload Changes: One new change will be to complete one of the exercises from the circuit twice in one set for all three sets (repeat one exercise) – for example spend 80 seconds doing squats instead of 40 and still have a rest like it's just another exercise. Also remember to keep training 40 seconds per exercise.

**Thursday –** Rest Day

**Friday –**

What to Train: High Impact Circuit 1

Progressive Overload Changes: Add 10 seconds to each exercise, you will either be training for 40 seconds or 70 seconds.

**Saturday –**

What to Train: High Impact Circuit 2

Progressive Overload Changes: Add 10 seconds to each exercise, you will either be training for 40 seconds or 70 seconds.

**Sunday –** Rest Day.


**Week 3 Overview:**

This week goes hard! I have now introduced progressive overload to both high impact circuits by increasing the exercise duration. I have doubled up on progressive overload for the medium impact circuit, meaning you should always exercise for 40 seconds at a time and repeat an exercise for each set. This week included around 130 minutes of exercise.


**Week 4**

**Monday –**

What to Train: High Impact Circuit 1

Progressive Overload Changes: No new changes, remember the previous changes and apply them to your circuit.

**Tuesday –** Rest Day

**Wednesday –**

What to Train: Medium Impact Circuit

Progressive Overload Changes: No new changes.

**Thursday –**

What to Train: High Impact Circuit 2

Progressive Overload Changes: No new changes

**Friday –**

What to Train: High Impact Circuit 1

Progressive Overload Changes: No new changes

**Saturday –**

What to Train: Medium Impact Circuit

Progressive Overload Changes: Now train this circuit at 75% of your Max HR – this will make you get a greater sweat on. Don't forget that the previous changes still apply.

**Sunday –** Rest Day

**Week 4 Overview:**

You may look at this week and think there are no new changes apart from the progressive overload change to the medium circuit which will make you train harder. The main change you should notice is that there are now 5 training days, this will allow you to reach roughly 165 minutes of weekly exercise. Keep it going, make sure to focus on recovery as there are only two rest day from now on.

## Week 5

**Monday –**

What to Train: High Impact Circuit 2

Progressive Overload Changes: No new changes from last week.

**Tuesday –** Rest Day

**Wednesday –**

What to Train: Medium Impact Circuit

Progressive Overload Changes: No new changes from last week – still apply previous changes.

**Thursday –**

What to Train: High Impact Circuit 1

Progressive Overload Changes: Start training the high impact circuits at 80% of your Max HR. Still apply the extra 10 second exercise period. Can be done by completing more reps in the 40 second period.

**Friday –**

What to Train: High Impact Circuit 2

Progressive Overload Changes: Train at 80% of Max HR and train each exercise for 40/70 seconds.

**Saturday -**

What to Train: High Impact Circuit 1

Progressive Overload Changes: No new changes – train just how you did on Thursday.

**Sunday –** Rest Day

**Week 5 Overview:**

A tough week. The progressive overload changes include an increase in intensity to 80% to make it harder for you. All the circuits are now at the highest difficult due to the changes, of course you can make them harder yourself after the last week. This week includes 165 minutes of exercise.

**Week 6 – Final Week**

**Monday –**

What to Train: High Impact Circuit 2

Progressive Overload Changes: No new changes.

**Tuesday –** Rest Day

**Wednesday –**

What to Train: High Impact Circuit 1

Progressive Overload Changes: No new changes

**Thursday –**

What to Train: High Impact Circuit 2

**Friday –**

What to Train: HIIT Circuit Taster

Progressive Overload Changes: No new changes.

**Saturday –**

What to Train: Initial Medium Impact Circuit

Progressive Overload: Only for this day train the medium impact circuit but train it how you were on the 1st week.

**Sunday –** Rest Day. The last day of the six-week plan but not your last day of training.

## Six-Week Overview:

Firstly, I want to congratulate you on getting this far. It is a real achievement to try something new and stick to it. I hope that you notice positive changes with your body, and you are in a great training routine now of exercising 5 days a week.

This is the only week where I include the HIIT taster circuit, this is a harder circuit so that is one of the ways I have implemented progressive overload. Another way I increased the difficulty was by increasing the length of the exercise period – this also means you exercise 150+ minutes a week.

I have included the taster HIIT circuit to give you an insight to what it is like so you can make the decision to read the last book of this series. I have avoided reducing the rest time with the progressive overload changes because I want everyone to get at least 150 minutes of moderate exercise in a week. But you must remember to not stop training after this.

You have all the information, resources and examples that will allow you to carry on training each week. Remember to use progressive overload to increase the difficulty of the circuit over time, allow yourself enough rest and you can reach your goals. If you reach your goal after a certain period then you will have to keep training to maintain your goal, when you reach this you can continue training each week but just refrain from making it harder. Surpassing your goal for weight loss may not be the best thing as you can easily get to an underweight stage, which you will have to then focus on gaining weight (Reversing progress).

You can take your fitness journey in any direction, it is common for people to start building muscle after losing weight to fill the hole in a positive way. This series won't be helpful for you building muscle but the HIIT circuits can help you shred down to get the perfect physique – this is just an option of course. If you don't enjoy training 5 days a week then go back to four but make sure you train longer on those days. It really is now up to you.

# Chapter 8 – The Exercise Descriptions You Need to Ace Your Workouts

You can find a description for every single exercise listed in this book within this chapter. The exercise descriptions are in order of which the circuits show them and will also be under the title for the specific circuit(s) they appear in.

### Medium Impact Exercises

**Jogging on the Spot** – Light run on the spot, just transfer weight from one leg to the other repeatedly. No picture included because c'mon everyone knows how to jog on the spot.

**Russian Twists** - Start in a sitting position so that your body and upper legs are in a "V" shape, to do this sit up on the floor while slightly leaning back, have your knees slightly raised and bent (1st photo). Start on the left side by holding your hands together next to your left hip, use your core and lower back to twist your body from left to right and use your hands to tap the floor either side of your body. Tap from left to right, right to left for the time given. Cross your ankles if you feel it helps you balance. This exercise strengthens obliques, abdominals and lower back.

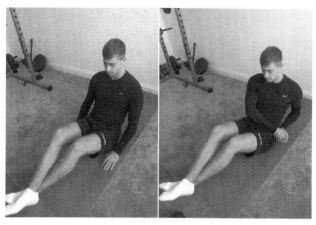

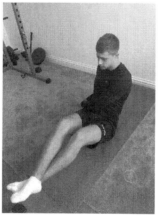

**Lunges with twists-** Start by standing with legs shoulder-width apart, then take a big step with your left foot forwards and bend your knees into it, you will feel the stretch and then proceed to use your back to twist your torso to the left then to the right before stepping back. Then step forwards with your right foot and twist your torso left to right. Continue to swap legs and this exercise is great for strengthening legs.

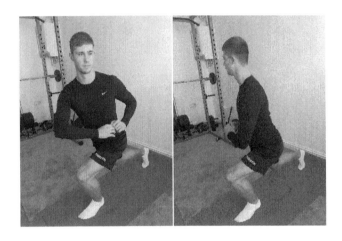

**Straight Punches** – Start by standing in a causal boxing stance, do this by placing your weak foot (pointing forwards) in front of your strong foot (facing outwards) with your arms held high and fists clenched like the 1st photo shows below – always keep your knees slightly bent. To throw a left straight punch then simply extend your left arm out quickly until you cannot extend your arm anymore, which then you should instantly bring your arm back to the starting position – always keep a clenched fist and the punch should be like a snap. To throw a right straight punch, follow the same steps as the left straight punch but twist your body while the punch is thrown. My boxing book can always help you with form. The benefits from this include faster hands, will make you sweat and potentially improve hand eye coordination. Repeat left-right-left-right straight punches for the time period.

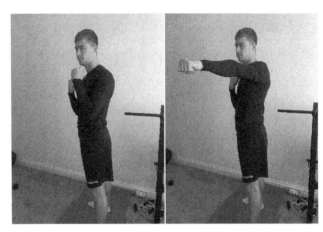

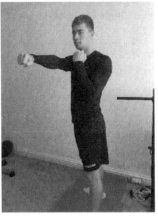

**Lying Superman Hold** – Starting position: Picture 1 shows that you should lay down facing the floor with your arms slightly in front of you bent and your legs slightly apart while relaxed.

Then use your core and back to raise your arms and legs off the ground, hold this position for a second or two before relaxing your muscles back into the starting position. Continue this for 30 seconds, a great core exercise.

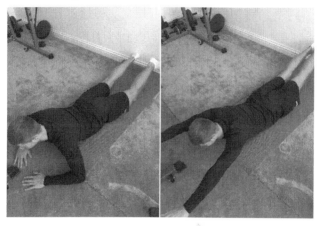

**Tuck Jumps** – From the usual standing position bend your knees slightly and push through your heels to jump up into the air, once your feet have left the ground tuck your knees into your chest by bending them. Be careful as you need to prepare for the impact of your fall so don't spend too long in the tuck position. This exercise will build up power in your leg muscles, along with help you burn fat and allow you to get worn out quickly. Don't worry about trying to jump as high as dec here!

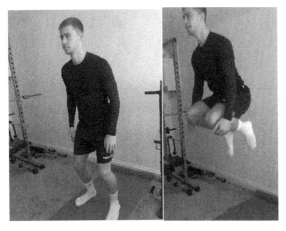

**Crunches** – Start by laying on the floor facing the sky with your arms crossed over your chest. Bring your knees up and make sure your feet are together while planted on the floor. From this starting position use your core and lower back to bring your chest about halfway to your knees, once you reach this point slowly release and lower yourself back to the ground. Complete as many as you can in the time, this will let you build up abs and burn belly fat.

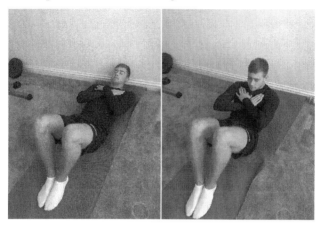

**Squats** –Start with feet shoulder-width apart and pointing outwards. Put weight into your heels, sit your bum back and bend your knees to lower yourself until your thighs are almost parallel to the floor, from this position push up through your heels to complete a squat. Keep your arms out in front of you while doing this to improve balance and avoid this exercise if you have knee problems. This exercise is brilliant for building stronger legs.

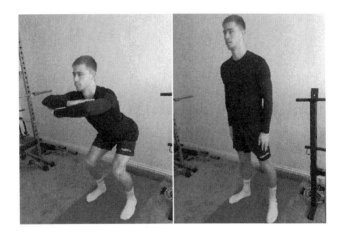

**High Impact Circuit 1 Exercises**

**Run on the spot** – A slightly faster pace than the light jog on the spot. No picture attached due to the simplicity of the activity.

**Knee to chest Taps** – Begin by standing with knees slightly bent and feet shoulder-width apart facing slightly outwards. Then proceed to tap your knees with your hands, make sure to keep your back straight and bend your knees while doing this, then slightly straighten your legs and tap your chest. Keep on tapping your knees then your chest on repeat for the time required. Tap at a fast pace because you are working at a higher intensity. If you are bending your knees correctly then you will start to feel it in your calves and quads, meaning this exercise will improve muscular endurance in your legs as well as burn fat.

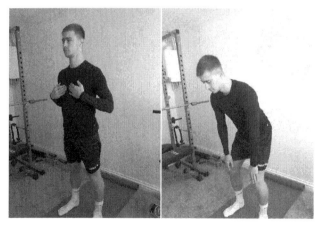

**Calf Raise** – Start in the usual standing position but be on your tiptoes. Simply press up through your tiptoes slowly as high as you can go, once you reach that position slowly lower your heels to the floor. Continue to repeat that motion slowly to feel the burning sensation in your lower legs. This exercise is brilliant for strengthening your calves, usually done by holding weights or on the edge of a stool however this book requires no equipment and it still allows you to feel the burn when doing them on a flat surface.

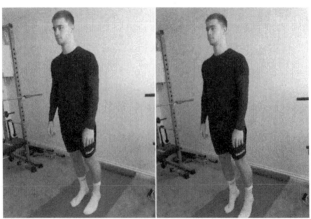

**Squat Jumps** – Firstly stand with your feet slightly wider than shoulder width apart and facing outwards. Then squat down by sitting back and shifting your weight into your heels while bending your knees, once you get as low down as you can, push up through your heels to jump up explosively. Use your arms to help create momentum for your jump. Once you land the squat jump you should carry on going until your times up! Great for building strength mainly in quads, hamstrings, calves, glutes as well as lower back muscles and abdominals. Requires many different muscles to perform a jump meaning you will burn calories and improve explosive power.

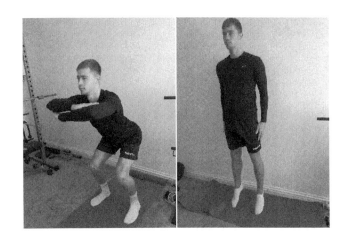

**Left to Right Jabs** – Start by standing with your knees slightly bent, feet facing outwards and your fists raised like the 1st photo shows below. Start on the left side by slightly bending your knees, then twisting your body to the left and throwing a jab with your left hand (2nd photo). After the jab is thrown pull your hands back into a boxer guard, then twist your torso from left to right while slightly squatting to which you should throw a jab with your right. Continue to jab left then right for the time, this exercise will improve your agility and make you sweat.

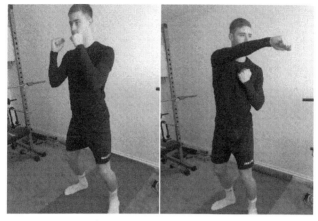

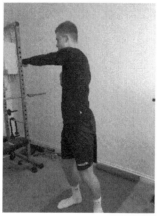

**Ali Shuffle** – Start with your left foot in front of your right and knees slightly bent. Then hop off the ground slightly so you can bring your left foot back and your right foot forwards at the same time, then you land you should hop again and then shuffle your feet back to the starting position. Do this continuously so you are always swapping feet. A great cardiovascular activity that will improve foot-eye coordination and will give you fast feet. (If you have ankle weights knocking about then stick them on!) This exercise was made popular by the great Muhammed Ali and look how it helped him out.

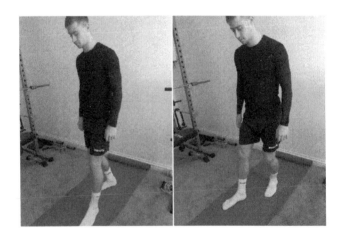

**Pushups** – Start in the position which the 1st photo shows, to do then place hands on the floor underneath your shoulders with your arms extended and have your legs straight with your tiptoes holding you up. Use your arms to lower your chest so that it almost touches the floor then from that position push up to get back to the starting position to complete a rep. Do as many reps as you can in the time, if you are new to pushups then complete them slowly with good form to get the hang of it. Pushups are great for strengthening triceps, pectorals (chest) and deltoid (shoulders). Pushups can be completed in many ways to improve endurance and train other certain muscles as well.

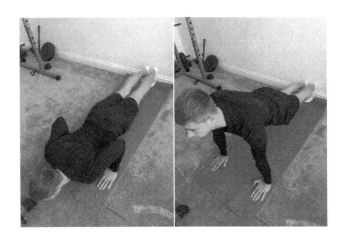

**Squat and Hamstrings** – This is more like a sequence of two exercises which work a treat together to wear you out. The sequence contains two squats then two hamstring kick-ups (one left, one right). Begin by standing with feet slightly wider than shoulder width apart, knees slightly bent and feet facing outwards. Then complete 2 quick squats by sitting back and bending your knees and pushing up through your heels, after that stand back up to which you want to kick your left foot back and up towards your bum while leaning slightly to the left and repeat with your right foot – make sure you lean to each side. This is a fun exercise that works your quads, abs, glues, calves and hamstrings.

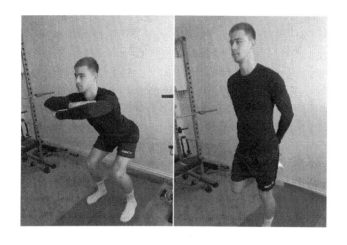

**Marching Air Punches** – Start by marching on the spot – very easy just lift your left knee then right knee in alternative order like you are walking with high knees. However, every time that your lift your left leg up you should punch straight up with your right hand, therefore when your right leg is raised you will punch up with your left hand. Continue to switch hands and legs for the time given, this is effectively an entire body workout which will build endurance in your arms and legs.

## High Impact Circuit 2 Exercises

**Left to Right Jabs** – Previously explained. A good cardiovascular activity to start the circuit.

**Lateral Split Squats** – Stand with your feet wide apart and your knees slightly bent, you can also choose to hold your hands out in front to maintain balance. Lean to your left so that most of your weight is on your left leg and bend your left knee to lower your body while keeping your right leg straight. Once you have lowered your body as far as you can slowly push up with your left leg then transfer your weight to your right leg and then bend into your right knee while keeping your left leg straight. This should feel like squatting on your left leg then your right. Repeat this for the time given. This targets your glutes, quads and inner thighs. While also improving flexibility.

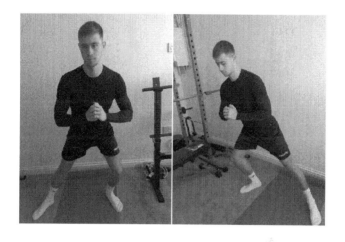

**Left, Right Floor Taps** - Start by standing with legs slightly bent and feet pointing slightly outwards. Keep hands by your side in the starting position, reach down with your left hand and tap the floor to the left of your left foot, stand back up and repeat this but tap the right side of your right foot with your right hand. Continue this motion for the time given. Remember to bend your legs when bending down to avoid back injuries.

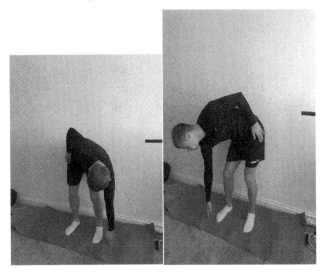

**Forwards and Back Crawl** – Start with hands and feet planted on the floor like how the 1st photo shows below, your hands in this position. Always have your feet planted in the same position while doing this. Crawl forwards by lifting and placing your left-hand forwards like the 2nd photo shows, then follow up with your right hand to get into the pushup position of photo 3. From the final position reverse the steps to crawl back to the position of photo 1. Continue to crawl back and forwards for the time given to get a sweat on, strengthen your arms and your core.

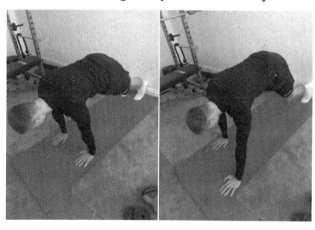

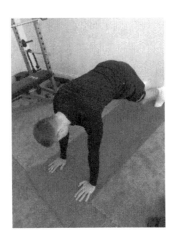

Side Lunges- Begin by standing light on your feet with feet slightly apart. Lunge left by stepping as far as you can left with your left foot and bend your left knee into it. Keep your right leg straight, your feet should always face outwards and always face forwards. From that position keep your feet planted to the ground, lean to the right side and switch your legs so that your left leg is now straight, and your right leg is bent. Continue to switch from side to side, this exercise will work your core, quads and glutes. The pictures below should help. These are different to lateral split squats because you don't have to get as low down for these and can be completed quicker to keep a higher heart rate.

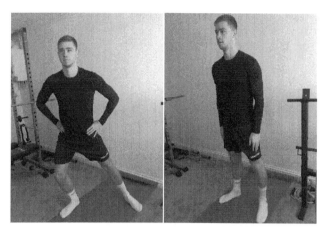

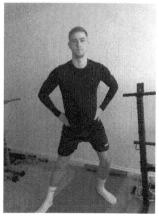

**High Knee Twists** – Start by standing with feet shoulder width apart. Start on left side, bring your left knee to your chest while using your arms and lower back to twist your torso to the left, as you bring your knee back down twist your torso back to normal position. Repeat this but lift your right knee up and twist your body to the right. Carry on in the sequence of left high knee to right high knee for the time given. This exercise will strengthen lower back and obliques, if completed at a good tempo then will your keep heart rate high.

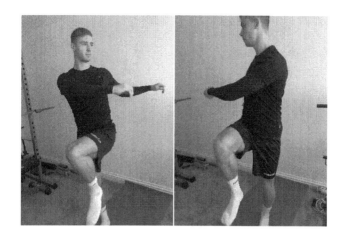

**Wide Push-Ups** - Start in the Wide Push Up Stance (Shown in the 1st picture), to get to this position lay face down on the floor with your legs together and extended while keeping your hands planted on the floor either side of your shoulders, simply push up and stay on your tip toes to get into the stance shown on the left. To complete a wide pushup simply just lower your chest to the floor and push back up using your arms. This particular push up targets your pectoral muscles along with triceps and shoulders, this is harder than a standard pushup meaning your muscles will get stronger.

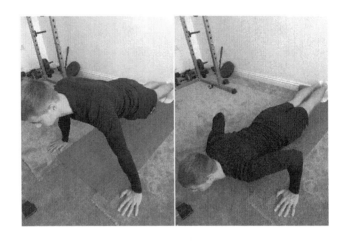

**Heel Flicks** – Another great cardiovascular activity. Start by standing up straight with feet shoulder width apart, put your hands over your bum and stay light on your feet (Keep heels off the floor). Start with your left leg by kicking back with your left foot, aim to kick your bum and then bring your foot back down. After you have raised and lowered your left leg, you should do the same with your right. Keep flicking your feet, left then right, for the time given.

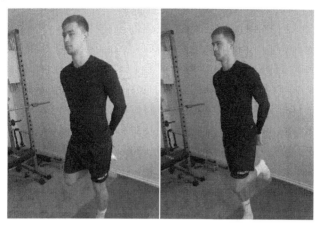

**Plank-** Begin by laying on the floor facing the floor and keep your forearms flat on the ground underneath your chest along with the rest of your body. To get into the plank push up slightly with your forearms and your feet so that the only parts of your body connecting with the floor are your arms and tiptoes. Hold this position for the time given if you can. This exercise is fantastic for our entire body, but most importantly burns belly fat and strengthens abs. The photo below shows the plank in action, don't raise your bum too high while planking as that is cheating, you should feel the burn while planking.

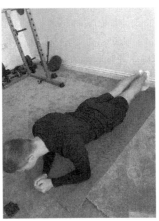

**Other Exercises**

Here are other exercises that are included in this book, however, don't fit into the main "Impact" circuits.

**Boxer Squat** – Begin by standing with feet facing slightly outwards and place feet wider than shoulder width apart. Keep your hands up in a boxer guard like shown in the 1st photo. Squat down by sitting back and bending your knees as far down as you can go. Then from the squat position push up through your heels back to the starting position and throw a straight left and a straight right punch (1-2). To punch extend your arms your quickly in front of you one after the other then bring your arms back to the starting boxer guard position to go again.

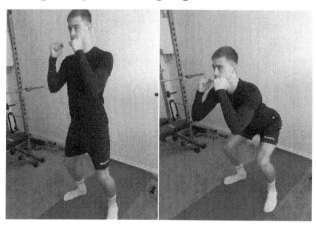

**Standing Side Hops** – Start by standing with feet and legs together and arms down by your sides. Then lean to the left, slightly bend your legs to jump up while keeping both feet together and land slightly to the left – use your hips to move while in the air. To hop to the right, lean to the right, bend knees to jump up and use your hips to move your feet to the right. In a quick motion, hop from left to right then right to left on repeat for the time given. Will mainly strengthen your calves and is heavily cardio based.

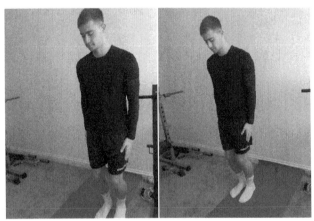

**Twist Jumps** – Stand with feet slightly wider than shoulder width apart, drop into a squat while twisting your body and arms to the left. Then quickly swing your arms to the right to and use your lower back to twist your torso to the right while jumping up through your heels so that you rotate 90 degrees clockwise in the air. Land the jump and repeat, change direction after 15 seconds. Improves agility, flexibility in hips and leg strength.

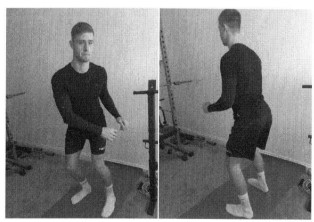

**Standing Side Crunch** – Begin by standing straight with your hands behind your head with fingers locked together. Use your hands to push your head down to the left while leaning to the left and raising your left knee (2nd photo), this should make you feel a slight burn in you obliques. Hold that position for a second before lowering your left leg, then lean to the right and raise your right knee to feel the same burn just this time on the other side (3rd photo). This exercise helps your improve balance and strengthen obliques.

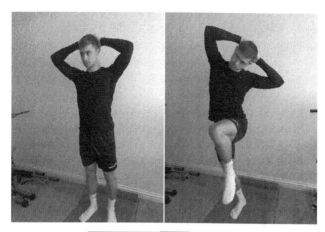

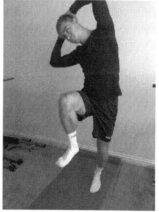

**Ankle Taps** – Begin by laying down on the floor facing the sky. Keep your arms by your sides as you need to mainly use your arms in this exercise. Your feet should be planted on the floor.

To complete an ankle tap: Reach for your left ankle with your left hand and try to touch your ankle, remember to stay in the initial laying position. Afterwards, bring your left hand back while reaching out to tap to your right ankle with your right hand. This exercise is great for strengthening obliques. Continue to tap both ankles for the time given.

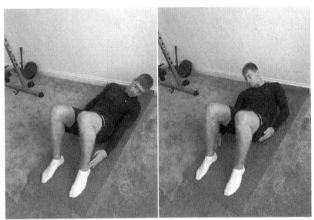

**Warmup Exercises**

**Marching on the spot** – From a standing position, lift your left knee about halfway to your chest, then lower your left foot to the ground before lifting your right knee then lower again. Continue to repeat this slowly to get the heart pumping.

**Arm circles** – Start by standing tall and bring your arms out straight on either side so that you are shaped like a capital "T". Imagine that you are drawing circles with your fingers, start by drawing small circles then slowly make your circles bigger. You will be using your shoulders to get the circular motion in your arms, switch direction after 15 seconds.

**Left Right Floor Taps** – Find the description earlier on in this chapter. Complete at a very light intensity for 60 seconds.

**Quad Stretch** – This requires a good level of balance so try to get something sturdy to lean on. Start standing in the usual position. Bring your left heel to your bum and hold it there with your left hand, use your right hand to lean on a sturdy object and hold this for 10-15 seconds. Swap to your right leg afterwards.

**Cross-body Shoulder Stretch** – Can be done standing or sitting. Start with your left shoulder: Bring your extended left arm across your torso so your left hand is past your right shoulder. With your right wrist, you want to press on your left wrist towards you so that you feel the burn in your left shoulder. Repeat this but follow the steps alternatively to stretch your right shoulder. Hold this for 10-15 seconds each arm.

**Chest Expansion** – Dynamic Stretch. Start by standing straight with your arms extended in front of you together like you have just clapped. Keep arms extended, separate your arms and bring them back as far as you can until your chest is puffed out. Hold that position for a second before bringing your arms forwards and your hands together. This should be done all in one motion, keep repeating for 30 seconds.

**Jog on Spot** – Hopefully it's not worth me explaining this aha… Just like you are running but not in any direction.

**Knee Hugs** – From a standing position, raise your left knee to your chest and hold it for a few seconds before letting go and swapping to perform the hug with your right leg. Continue to repeat this for 30 seconds.

**Sexy Circles** – Stand tall with your feet wide apart and keep your hands on your hips. For the 30 seconds, proceed to rotate your hips in circles using your legs and lower back to do so. This exercise loosens up your hips and groin, remember to spend 15 seconds going clockwise, 15 seconds anti-clockwise and make sure you look good doing it!

**Arm Extension Hold** – In a standing or sitting position, raise both arms up as high as you can and lock your fingers together. From that position roll your shoulders up to extend your arms further and push up through your fingers, hold this for 10-15 seconds to give your arms a good stretch then you should stretch again after a slight rest. Overall, stretch twice in the 30 second period.

**Ankle Rolls** – Stand with feet shoulder width apart. Raise your left heel so that your tiptoes are on the floor and have your right foot planted, then rotate your left ankle clockwise using your tiptoes. After 15 or so seconds, switch foot so your right foot is on its tiptoes then rotate for 15 seconds. This stretches the ligaments, muscles and tendons.

**Lateral Split Squat Stretch** – This is previously explained as an exercise. However, this time you should complete the Lateral Split Squats slowly so that you feel the stretch. This means that every time you squat to the left or right you should hold it for 5 or so seconds before returning to a standing position. Continue to stretch each side on and off for 30 seconds. This stretches most of the major leg muscles.

**High Kick Outs** – This requires lots of space to complete. From a standing position you will need to kick out in front of you with your left leg while your right foot is planted, try to get your left leg as high as you can while keeping it extended. Once your foot gets as high as you can bring your left leg down and repeat the kick out

371

with your right leg. Continue to kick and swap legs for the 30 seconds. This yet again stretches leg muscles and uses your core.

**Heel Flicks** – Previously Explained, just this time complete sat a slower rate for a minute to raise your heart rate and get you ready for the circuits.

## Cooldown Exercises

**Shake off Body** – Start with your legs, just lift one foot off the floor at a time to shake it off then move on to the arms which you can shake off one at a time.

**Side to Side** – From a standing position with your hands down by your sides, slowly lower your left hand until you reach your left knee – at the same time your torso should be bending to the left and your right hand should be raised to your chest area. Hold that position for a couple seconds before slowly raising your left hand and lowering your right hand until it reaches your right knee. This will stretch your back, shoulders and core.

**Forward Fold** – Stand straight with feet wide apart, bend your body forwards while keeping your back straight and reach down towards the floor. Hold this position for a few seconds before getting back up, resting for a short moment then going again.

**Open the Gates** – Previously explained, however this time just rotate your hips slowly while opening the gates.

**Cross Body Shoulder Stretch** – In a standing or sitting position, bring our left arm across your chest as far as you can reach, then use your right forearm to hold that stretch for 10 to 15 seconds. After that repeat with the other arm by reaching across your chest with your right arm then push that arm towards your chest with your left forearm to stretch the shoulders and triceps.

**Side Leg Raises** – Begin by laying down on your side with your left leg to the floor. Then you will need to slowly raise your right foot in the air while keeping your left leg stationary across the floor, continue to raise and lower your right leg for 15 seconds before rolling over so that your right leg is laying across the floor. In this position raise and lower your left leg for 15 seconds. This dynamic stretch works your outer thighs.

# Chapter 9 – Training Towards Greatness

I have done my part, so now it's time to do yours. You now have all the information, motivation, circuits, exercises and much more in one book so you can get into a great training routine. If this book wasn't enough for you then you have the other two books from this series to read and take information from, if you haven't come from the beginner's book and find these circuits very challenging then I suggest that you have a read of "Circuit Training for Beginners". Or if you are interested in taking your training further then I can suggest "High Intensity Circuit Training".

There are so many routes you can take with your fitness journey, whether it's training to gain muscle mass, training to become stronger, training to improve endurance and many more training routines. I suggest training to gain muscle mass because that will help you keep at a healthy weight after losing all the fat, yet again it is all up to you. If you continue to keep exercising and eat well then, I do not have a problem. You can of course join a gym, start joining clubs like boxing or football, the possibilities are endless.

"High Intensity Circuit Training" is the final book of this series, this book can also act as a standalone, but it makes sense to read after reading the other two books. HIIT stands for High Intensity Interval Training, this is a cardiovascular exercise strategy that alternates short periods of intense anaerobic exercise with less intense recovery periods. To put it simply, this will include a short period of very hard exercise followed by a short rest – the very hard exercise should leave you gasping for breath as you are giving it your all. HIIT circuits are great for those looking to burn fat while keeping their muscle mass high, as longer periods of moderate exercise tend to burn more muscle along with fat opposed to HIIT. The best thing about HIIT in my opinion is that it can be done anywhere with no equipment, so hopefully that has given you a good insight to the next book.

# Conclusion

Thank you for making it to the end of Intermediate Circuit Training and I hope that you enjoyed reading and learning along the way. Whether you have read the first two books of the series or this is the only book you plan to read I am still grateful for you giving me a chance. You should be able to get some great workouts in at home now and stick to a fun workout routine. My advice is to complete these home circuits regularly if you are interested in just losing weight and change up your current diet if you are not getting all the nutrients required – this is most likely going to end up with you saving money as gyms can be pricey compared to these home workouts which are free. Obviously, it is up to you where you take your fitness journey, I would only suggest joining a gym if you will be looking to build muscle as buying individual weights are expensive and may require maintenance. But don't always look to continue to lose weight as you will have nothing left to lose eventually which is unhealthy and most importantly always have a goal you can work towards.

To conclude this book, here is a brief summary chapter by chapter to refresh your memory. Chapter 1 starts with a recap of the first book of the series which covers the basics of diet, circuit training, training zones, equipment and an example circuit for the new readers so they understand this book without having to read others. Chapter 2 is all about helping you develop the winning mindset which helps you stick to your training routine as well as being helpful to make you determined and confident with many things in life – I believe balance to be very important. The third chapter covers diet in detail, this includes information about the essential nutrients and what food contains them, information about what makes up a healthy diet, the benefits that come with a great diet and finally a day's diet plan which acts as an example for you to structure your diet plan on.

Moving on to chapter 4 which focuses on warmups, cooldowns, resting, recovery and recovery tips which all influence preparation for recovery. Chapter 5 which goes over components of exercising and many tips and tricks to help you exercise to your max potential which will allow you to reach your goals quicker. Chapter 6 is the main chapter that includes 8 circuits which can all be trained at home – each circuit contains information on how it will help you, but they all are under the category of weight loss. Chapter 7, another big chapter, contains the six-week plan that is where you can get into a great fitness routine and learn how to use progressive overload to improve your fitness levels.

Chapter 8 is a chapter filled with exercise descriptions with picture examples that link to the exercises used in the circuits. This covers all exercises in the book, even the exercises found in the warmups and cooldowns. Finally, you reach chapter 9, a chapter with the title What's Next? Well, this chapter discusses the possibilities of where you can take your fitness journey after this book, I give a few options, but my main goal is to persuade you to actually stick to training and not let it slip. That's all from me, Thank you. It really is a pleasure that you are allowing me to persuade your fitness journey and I am sure it will benefit you.

# References

*Dec Beales - Model for the Exercise*

*Demonstrations.*

https://www.instagram.com/dec.beales/

*Your Free Gift – The Circuit Training Weight Loss*

*Bundle.*

*https://hudsonandrew.activehosted.com/f/33*

*Join the Facebook Community.*

https://www.facebook.com/groups/workoutf

orweightloss

*Follow my Facebook Page.*

https://www.facebook.com/andrewhudsonbooks1

*Email me for extra support.*

andrew@hudsonandrew.com

A.H. (2020a). *Benefits of Exercise*. AH. https://medlineplus.gov/benefitsofexercise.html#:~:text=Exercise%20strengthens%20your%20heart%20and,blood%20pressure%20and%20triglyceride%20levels.

A.H. (2020b). *Breathing*. AH. https://blog.nasm.org/the-right-way-to-breathe-during-exercise#:~:text=The%20gold%20standard

%20during%20strength,ramps%20up%2C%20through%20the%20mouth.

A.H. (2020c). *Caffeine Benefits*. AH. https://time.com/4842065/coffee-before-workout-caffeine/#:~:text=Caffeine%20can%20shift%20muscles%20to,its%20efficiency%20in%20generating%20power.

A.H. (2020d). *Diabetes*. AH. https://www.helpguide.org/articles/diets/the-diabetes-diet.htm#:~:text=Limit%20refined%20carbohydrates%20like%20white,from%20producing%20too%20much%20insulin.

A.H. (2020e). *Exercise motivation.* AH. https://intermountainhealthcare.org/blogs/topics/live-well/2018/05/5-tips-for-exercise-motivation/

A.H. (2020f). *Fiber benefits.* AH. https://www.healthline.com/nutrition/why-is-fiber-good-for-you#TOC_TITLE_HDR_3

A.H. (2020g). *Getting into a routine:* AH. https://www.nm.org/healthbeat/healthy-tips/health-benefits-of-having-a-routine#:~:text=Routines%20Can%20Be%20Fun&text=Better%20stress%20levels%20lead%20to,to%20relax%20and%20less%20anxiety.&text=Your%20sleep%20schedule%

20and%20bedtime,waking%20and%20goin
g%20to%20bed.

A.H. (2020h). *Good v. Bad carbs*. AH.
https://my.clevelandclinic.org/health/articles
/15416-
carbohydrates#:~:text=Good%20carbs%20ta
ke%20longer%20to,mainly%20white%20flo
ur%20and%20sugar

A.H. (2020i). *Healthy Breakfast*. AH.
https://www.mayoclinic.org/healthy-
lifestyle/nutrition-and-healthy-eating/in-
depth/food-and-nutrition/art-20048294

A.H. (2020j). *How food affects the brain*.
AH. https://blog.genomind.com/how-food-

can-affect-your-

brain#:~:text=Our%20brains%20function%
20best%20when,which%20can%20damage
%20brain%20cells.

A.H. (2020k). *Importance of Fats*. AH.

https://www.heart.org/en/healthy-

living/healthy-eating/eat-smart/fats/dietary-

fats#:~:text=Dietary%20fats%20are%20esse

ntial%20to,Your%20body%20definitely%20

needs%20fat.

A.H. (2020l). *Importance of protein +*
*carbs*. AH.

https://www.nia.nih.gov/health/important-

nutrients-know-proteins-carbohydrates-and-

fats

A.H. (2020m). *Lung Capacity*. AH.

https://www.healthline.com/health/how-to-

increase-lung-capacity


A.H. (2020n). *Meal Tips*. AH.

https://healthmaxphysio.com/spacing-meals-

4-simple-

tips/#:~:text=Research%20shows%20that%

20spacing%20out,a%20decrease%20in%20e

nergy%20expenditure.


A.H. (2020o). *Mineral deficiency*. AH.

https://www.healthline.com/health/mineral-

deficiency

A.H. (2020p). *Minerals*. AH.
https://www.dailymail.co.uk/femail/article-8204/Minerals-15.html

A.H. (2020q). *More exercise benefits*. AH.
https://greatist.com/fitness/13-awesome-mental-health-benefits-exercise#productivity

A.H. (2020r). *Over Motivation*. AH.
https://thesquashcompany.com/dangers-motivated-part-i/#:~:text=Like%20too%20much%20of%20anything,situation%20harder%20to%20turn%20around.

A.H. (2020s). *Problems with over-exercising:* AH.

_https://medlineplus.gov/ency/patientinstructi_
_ons/000807.htm_

A.H. (2020t). *Rest and Recovery*. AH.
https://www.verywellfit.com/ways-to-speed-
recovery-after-exercise-3120085

A.H. (2020u). *Stress Advice*. AH.
https://www.mayoclinic.org/healthy-
lifestyle/stress-management/in-
depth/exercise-and-stress/art-
20044469#:~:text=Exercise%20increases%2
0your%20overall%20health,%2Dgood%20n
eurotransmitters%2C%20called%20endorph
ins.

A.H. (2020v). *Tips to boost mental health*. AH. https://www.mhanational.org/31-tips-boost-your-mental-health

A.H. (2020w). *Vitamins*. AH. https://www.medicalnewstoday.com/articles/195878

A.H. (2020x). *Water*. AH. https://www.efbw.org/index.php?id=46#:~:text=Water%20carries%20nutrients%20to%20all,helps%20to%20regulate%20body%20temperature

# High Intensity Circuit Training

*The New & Advanced Workout Routine for Burning Body Fat. Improve Your Fitness Levels, Develop a Determined Mindset, and Achieve Your Dream Body in 30 Days!*

## Andrew Hudson

# Introduction

"I have always got this fat on my belly that seems to never go away. It's always there when I look in the mirror, no matter what I do to try get rid of it, this stops me from having my perfect body and it's so frustrating. The perfect diet is so hard to commit to and I haven't got the time to train for longer. I just want to be able to get my body ready for summer and be proud about it."

This is part of a message that I received from a stranger, that stranger is now a good friend of mine and has been for many years, the reason that the connection was built because I helped her find a passion for living a healthy lifestyle so she could achieve her dream body. As a qualified personal trainer, I have helped many people in this situation and over the years I have been testing and researching the most effective ways for quick yet successful ways to burn fat.

After all the years of research and trying new training methods with my clients and myself, it has been clear to me that HIIT Circuits (A combination of High Intensity Interval Training and Circuit Training) is the most effective training methods to help lower body fat percentage and help people achieve their fitness goals. The best part is, HIIT Circuits can be set up in seconds, completed in under 30 minutes and requires no equipment! I love helping people reach their fitness goal because it lets them experience a range of benefits like an improved mental state, higher energy levels, a better body and much more that you will discover in this book.

You may ask, Andrew if you have found this successful method why are you writing and not coaching people? Well, as I have been stuck at home just like the millions of others, I think there is no better time to write as I can reach a larger number of people in a similar position to you. So that's what I do, I offer fitness help through my books to get people active at home instead of letting them lay on the sofa.

This book is much more than a few exercises written in a list. You will find nutritional information, a guide to the high protein diet, ways to enhance your training, how to go from training once a blue moon to training HIIT Circuits 5 days a week, 5 well-structured HIIT Circuits, motivational advice, meditation and a description for every exercise included in this book. Now that is something I wouldn't miss out on!

It's your turn to take action, however if you turn down this opportunity, although it's hard for me to say this, it is unlikely you will reach your fitness goals and please don't feel the need to live with regret. Instead, you should read this book now and start a new fitness routine as soon as you have finished reading. Exercising gets harder for every day you put it off, so start now! Just give it a real good go, if you can say you've given it a good go, but you didn't enjoy it then fair enough, it's the effort that counts.

## Circuit Training for Weight Loss

This is the last book from the three-part series, "Circuit Training for Weight Loss". This series is for people that are looking to reach fitness goals at home with the training method: Circuit Training. Whether your goal is to lose weight to meet job requirements, to improve your health or if you are looking to lower your body fat percentage to look ripped/toned then this series will help you out. Below you will find a brief description of each book and a summary of the series at the end, if you want to find out more, then search up the book titles to view the detailed description!

The first book of these series, it is the most basic, but that doesn't mean that you won't be able to lose weight from it! This book is to get you into a simple exercise routine, will help you clean up your diet and give you an understanding of general health and fitness. This book is a great starting point to set you off on your weight loss journey, helping you break your old unhealthy habits so you can no longer fall under the obese or overweight category.

The second book of the series, "Intermediate Circuit Training", is the next step that increases the difficulty of the workouts, so you make quicker progress towards harder fitness goals. This still sticks with the theme of weight loss with circuit training and nutrition, but this book starts to branch out to slightly more advanced health & fitness information and starts to present motivational advice, so you stay on track with your fitness goal. This isn't for complete beginners, more for the average person looking to lose weight.

The book you are now reading is the final book, "High Intensity Circuit Training", and is the most advanced book. The workouts in these books are shorter, but much more difficult and frequent as this book is to help people with difficult fitness goals like having a low body fat percentage and having a high lean muscle mass percentage. This book also offers advice on how to adapt your mindset to reach challenging goals, information about how to boost your metabolic rate and many other ways to burn fat quickly to lower your body fat percentage while building lean muscle mass. This is for the experienced fitness fanatics.

As you can see, each book from this series is like a steppingstone towards your final fitness goal. Each book goes up in difficulty and if you are looking to go from Fat to Fit, I highly recommend following each book 1 at a time to reach and maintain your goal of having your dream body!

# Your Free Gift

The Circuit Training Weight Loss Bundle is a combination of extras to help you reach your goals. These 'extras' can all help in their own way. Below are a few examples of what you may find in the bundle:

- An Equipment Checklist to help you find all the optional equipment that may help you with HIIT Circuits.

- A Calorie Tracking App that makes it very easy to split your diet up and keep on track of what you eat.

- An Extra HIIT Circuit – this one is what I call the Calisthenics HIIT Circuit.

- A Motivational Compilation filled with quotes, something to look at during struggle.

- A HIIT Circuit Cheat Sheet – This makes it easy to refer to the information provided. You may also find a couple other things hidden in the Circuit Training Weight Loss Bundle...

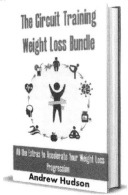

Follow this link to access the free eBook:

https://hudsonandrew.activehosted.com/f/33

# Join the Workout for Weight Loss Community

Living a healthy lifestyle is difficult, especially when you feel as if you are doing it all alone. That's why I suggest for you to join a community of others who are in your situation, this community "Workout for Weight Loss" will provide you with daily posts about weight loss and there will be many people that you can talk to, share experiences with and receive help from.

I aim to post twice a day, providing you with tips, tricks, motivation, workouts, diet plans and so much more to help you lose weight. Not to mention that I may host a few book giveaways every now and then. In a community, your chance of reaching your goals is much stronger and you may make many new friends in the process!

So, if you are looking for that extra help, please join my Free Facebook Group: https://www.facebook.com/groups/workoutforweightloss

# Chapter 1 – What is High Intensity Circuit Training?

**Who's This Book For?**

High Intensity Circuit Training is a training method that you probably haven't heard of before. HICT is just a mixture of Circuit Training and HIIT, both other these training methods you have probably heard of before. You will probably be able to tell from "High Intensity" that this book provides more advanced workouts for those that are looking to reach more difficult goals. More specifically, this book will help you lower your body fat percentage and gain lean muscle mass so that you look ripped as a man or toned as a woman.

Along your fitness journey you will of course experience many other benefits like improving your fitness level, building mental toughness and much more. So, there is much more than what meets the eye. So, I guess I could say this book is for health & fitness fanatics, although beginners will be able to read and follow this book, I strongly suggest for you to read the last two books of this series if you have less fitness experience.

Whether you want to lower your body fat percentage to look more toned/ripped, or if you want to become fitter because you are training for a certain event, or you just want to lose weight to fit into your favorite jeans. Any reason for wanting to burn fat is a good reason, the HIIT Circuits and advice in this book will help you along that journey. You will find plenty of advanced training advice and information which you can either implement to your HIIT Circuits or other types of training.

This book this the last one out of a three-part book series, the previous two books labelled "Circuit Training for Beginners" and "Intermediate Circuit

Training" both show that this book is the highest level of difficulty when it comes to exercise, meaning this will help those who have more extreme fitness goals and will make a real difference to your training routine. Furthermore, I suggest for those who are less experienced with exercising to check out my previous books of this series before giving this book a real go. That is just a suggestion, if you are a beginner but think HICT is the training type for you then give it a go for it and work towards completing a HIIT Circuit. (A HIIT Circuit is what I call the workouts in this book)

For most of the people reading, I guess you know your stuff when it comes to exercising, of course you can never know everything there is to know in a subject area because new information and research is being carried out each day by the professionals – what I am trying to say here is that I am still able to help you. You are at a level where you will be able to pick up information quickly and use that in your training routine. Even if you are at an average fitness level, you will have more to learn but don't be frightened by that just take it day by day at your own pace.

It is likely that you understand what HIIT is, and you understand how Circuit Training works, don't worry if you are clueless because it's covered in this book. It is likely that you also have a goal you want to reach that involves losing weight, yet again if you don't have a goal, I can help you make one. This book is just more than a Circuit Training guide, it goes much deeper into the mental side of training, provides many tips you can try to reach your fitness goals quicker, contains many facts on why HIIT Circuits are the best way to reach your goals, provides nutritional information and much more.

## Circuit Training Basics

Even if you exercise every day without an excuse, it is still possible that you don't know anything about Circuit Training, but I am sure that will soon change. Even if you do know a lot about Circuit Training as you have come from the previous books, I still suggest reading this to solidify your knowledge on the basics.

Circuit training is a workout technique that involves different exercises in a cycle with a rest in between each exercise. Circuits can have between 4 and 12 exercises in a cycle to really give you variety in what you train, there are many variables of the circuit that can be modified to suit you! The variables that make up circuit training and can be changed are:

- **Which Exercises to Include** - This can be any exercise from pushups to burpees, I have included many exercises in this book which require no equipment and can be done anywhere.

- **Number of Exercises in the Circuit** - How many exercises are in the circuit (for HIIT Circuits I suggest 6 to 10).

- **Number of Sets** - Completing a set is where you complete every exercise in the sequence for the required time, this means that if you complete the circuit twice then you've completed 2 sets.

- **Time Spent Doing Each Exercise** - How long you spend carrying out the exercise listed (I suggest around 20 seconds).

- **Time Spent Resting Between Exercises** - This is the valuable time you get for resting between exercises (I suggest 30 seconds).

- **Time Spent Resting Between Sets** - This is the time you have for resting between sets to catch your breath before starting another set (I suggest 1 or 2 minutes).

- **Intensity** - How hard you train (further explained in detail under subchapter intensity).

- **How Many Days a Week you Train** – The number of days a week that you complete a HIIT Circuit.

It is possible to change any variable – this allows for anybody (Beginner or Expert) to be able to complete a circuit as the difficulty of the circuit can be raised or lowered by changing certain variables that I will later explain which variables are the ones that you should change to make the workout more intense, so it becomes a HIIT Circuit. Below you can find a list of benefits associated with Circuit Training:

**Circuit Training is Time-Efficient:** The circuits in this book are very quick to set up and take around 20-30 minutes to complete.

**Circuit Training is Practical:** A circuit can be set up anywhere at any time, the circuits in this book require no equipment. Great for Home Workouts!

**Circuit Training has Variety:** You can fit absolutely any exercise into a circuit so that it allows you to train how you like, for example if you are looking to become stronger you can easily set up a circuit with certain exercises that will work certain muscles. You can also train with the exercises in a different order or train in different areas to provide variety to prevent boredom.

**Circuit Training is Easily Modified:** If you decide that the circuits provided aren't long enough then you can modify the circuit just by changing how long you spend on each exercise which will make the entire circuit longer.

**Circuit Training is for Anyone** – Can be done if you are any shape and size because it can be modified to suit you. I take consideration of any difficulties people may face (like joint problems) and I make circuits with exercises that don't require them to bend their joints. This book itself will not contain circuits modified for those with joint problems as they are too intense, refer to previous books. Plus, you will find advice to strengthen joints in this book.

**Circuit Training is Fun** – This method of training is much different to going on a run. It has a great range of exercises that will get you moving. You can always complete a circuit with another person, you can complete a circuit with music on or anything you like to make it enjoyable for you. If training is enjoyable then you are motivated.

## Example Circuit

Here is an example how the circuits are structured and described in this book. I start with listing a few instructions, the first one will be how many sets to complete. Secondly, I state how long to rest in between each exercise – please note that this not the same as the rest period between sets. Think of the rest between sets like Half-time in Soccer, it's a recovery period to prepare you to go again and this usually lasts 1 to 3 minutes. I may also word this as "Rest for 3 minutes after completing the first set". I then set you a target of what heart rate/training zone you should work at. I finally state the time it takes to complete the warmup, circuit and cooldown.

Complete 2 sets, rest for 30 seconds between each exercise with a 2-minute rest between each set. Train at the Light Training Zone

(Around 60% of Max HR). This circuit takes roughly 20 minutes to complete including the warmup and cooldown.

Warmup 4

13. Push-ups – 30 seconds

14. Marching on the spot – 30 seconds

15. Calf Raise – 30 seconds

16. Half Squats – 30 seconds

17. Knees to Chest – 30 seconds

18. Jog on the spot – 30 seconds

Cooldown 3

At the top and bottom of the circuit I include the phrase "Warmup 4" and "Cooldown 3", I have that there because it should remind you to warmup before the circuit and cooldown after the circuit.

"Warmup 4" is the name of a warmup I have provided in this book, you will need to be familiar with the warmups and cooldowns I provide in this book as you will be doing them before and after every circuit. If you are confused to where Warmup 1, 2 and 3 are then you would have to look back in the previous books because they suit easier circuits. (Although Warmup 3 is included in this book)

## Intensity

Intensity is an important variable that can be changed with ease to modify the difficulty of the training. The first two letters in HIIT stand for High Intensity, that is a big giveaway to how intense your Circuits should be. Before I tell you how hard you should be working, below are the training zones that will be used in this book. As you can see, each training zone is between two percentages of your max heart rate.

**Hard Training Zone** – 80-90% of max heart rate. You will be breathing heavily and working aerobically. At this intensity you are improving your speed endurance. Lactic Acid will be present in your blood, so training at this zone will allow for your body to handle it well, which will reduce cramps if you consistently train at this intensity. I do not recommend working in his zone for a long period as this may result in injury.

**Maximum** – 90-100% of max heart rate. Your body will be working at maximum capacity, you can only train in this zone for short periods of time as lactic acid builds up quickly in blood and can cause cramp or injury. The final circuit requires you to work at your Max Heart Rate, so please be careful while in this training zone and make sure to not overdo it.

To go into more detail, the reason why the training zones are determined by percentages of your max heart rate is because it makes the intensity specific to you. To prove my point, if I determined the intensity by asking for 20 jumping jacks in 30 seconds, people who are physically fitter will find that easier because their body has adapted to exercise over time – this means they will be working at a moderate intensity as their muscles don't need as much energy and nutrients that's supplied by blood to complete the 20 jumping jacks. On the other hand, people who aren't as fit will find it harder to complete the jumping jacks in the given time and their heart rate will higher, meaning they are working at a higher intensity.

You will need to be able to measure your max heart rate (HR) to find out what heart rates you should be working between for certain circuits. You can discover what your maximum heart rate is by subtracting your age from 220. For example, if you are 20 years old then you would have a max heart rate of 200bpm (200-20=200).

You will use your max heart rate to work out what heart rate you should be working between. I will use the light training zone as an example here. To find the lower percentage of the training zone (60% for light zone) you will have to divide your max heart rate by 100 and times that new number by 60 (200 / 100 = 2 X 60 = 120 bpm), next you will divide your max heart rate by 100, but times that number by 70 instead of 60 to find the higher percentage of the training zone (200/ 100 = 2 X 70 = 140bpm). If you are 20 years old and looking to work in the light training zone, then you will be lucky enough to have to work in between the nice round numbers of 120bpm and 140bpm.

## Why Train HIIT?

HIIT stands for High Intensity Interval Training. This means that the workout will contain short periods of intense and difficult exercise followed by a period of rest or easy and light exercise. Or to put it more professionally – A short work period followed by a slightly longer recovery period. Hopefully, you can already see how this can slide in perfectly with Circuit Training, but before I make the link between the two let's go deeper into HIIT.

HIIT should last no longer that 30 minutes, excluding the warmup and cooldown. This is because your body won't be able to cope with vigorous exercise for too long without risking injury – the recovery period allows you to catch your breath and slightly lower your heart rate to prevent your body overheating, muscles straining or just anything problematic with your body.

Below is a list of the Benefits that come with HIIT:

- HIIT can burn plenty of calories in a short amount of time – this is a massive benefit to those who don't have much time to exercise each day, you can get a brilliant workout in 20 to 30 minutes that will leave you sweating and burning plenty of calories. Researchers found that HIIT burns 20-30% more calories than other forms of exercise.

- Your Metabolic Rate is higher for hours after HIIT – This means that you will still be burning plenty of calories even a couple of hours after you exercise. Metabolism is later explained under the diet section, but I think it's the key for fat burning.

- HIIT can help you burn fat, that may be the most obvious benefit but consistently training HIIT will lower your body fat and the results will come faster than you think.

- You can build muscle with HIIT. That's right, even if you are looking to burn fat training HIIT will allow you to build an amazing physique underneath the layers of fat. The exercises provided in this book may all be body weight, however as you will be completing them at a level of near exhaustion, your muscles will have a harder time exerting and that will make it likely for them to rip and grow back bigger. You should be able to increase your lean muscle mass with HIIT.

- HIIT can improve oxygen consumption, this refers to how well your muscles can use oxygen. It usually takes a very long time of gradual increase of continuous training to increase your oxygen consumption, however it is proven that consistently completing HIIT can provide the same positive results to oxygen consumption in shorter period of time. So, your muscles will be using every bit of oxygen to the best of its ability.

- Can reduce Heart Rate and Blood Pressure – just like most exercise, consistent HIIT training will make you healthier. A lower resting heart rate is great because it shows that your heart is working well and pumping blood around the body efficiently. A lower blood pressure reduces the risk of stroke and kidney disease.

- Blood sugar can be reduced by HIIT and improves insulin resistance. This is very beneficial for those with Diabetes.

## Combining the Two

Adding HIIT and Circuit Training together leaves you with HIIT Circuits. These go hand in hand because you can set up your HIIT session in the style of how you can set up a circuit: let me explain further. HIIT Circuits = High Intensity Circuit Training.

If you look back at the sub-chapter "Circuit Training Basics", then you can see that circuit training is very flexible in the way you can train it because of all the variables that you can change. It is very simple to convert a low impact circuit to a high impact circuit by changing the variables – the variables such as intensity will need to be increased and time spent on exercise would need to be decreased. You can of course change other variables if you feel it contributes towards making the HIIT Circuit.

Just to make it clear, a HIIT Circuit requires around 6 to 10 exercises performed at a High Intensity (Above 80% of Max HR) with short periods of rest between exercises and sets. The reason you don't want to have too many exercises in the circuit is because it would most likely put the entire workout longer than 30 minutes and that can be dangerous.

The idea of a HIIT Circuit is to keep your heart pumping quickly for the duration of the Circuit to burn as many calories as you can, which helps you lower your body fat percentage. The HIIT Circuits provided have a large variety of exercises to keep it fun and motivating. A Gym Membership is not needed due to the No-Equipment Exercises meaning that you will save money, plus it saves you from having those embarrassing moments at the gym. Below is a list of benefits which I hope that will urge you to include HIIT Circuits in your training routine, most of these benefits are repeated but it's good to hear it again as it may motivate you more to start using HIIT Circuits.

- HIIT Circuits are time efficient – Under 30 minutes per HIIT Circuit.

- HIIT Circuits are easily set up – Mainly just requires an open space and a stopwatch
- HIIT Circuits are easily modified – There are many exercises and variables that can be changed to make the circuit suit you.
- HIIT Circuits get you into a routine – A key factor to keeping motivated.
- Doesn't have to be done alone – Makes it fun.
- Requires little to no equipment - No equipment is required; however, some equipment is optional as it may provide comfort or help towards your training.
- A real great home workout – If it is cold outside, or the gyms are shut then just find a bit of open space and get started.

HIIT is the most efficient training method to burn body fat. The short periods of intense exercise allow the body to burn calories efficiently without using muscles for energy which allow you to maintain your muscle mass. Longer exercise like continuous training requires more calories to be burned over a longer period and burns away small parts of your muscles to keep your body energized on a long training session. If you want to maintain your muscle mass, then stick to HIIT because the training sessions are shorter and don't rely on muscles for energy.

## Extra Information

Here you can find more information that links to HIIT, Circuit Training and so on. Like most things, there is always more than what meets the eye and I hope to have you including HIIT Circuits in your training routine.

HIIT is also a great training method to build lean muscle mass. Although this book isn't focused on bodybuilding or strength training, why wouldn't you want to build lean muscle mass? Firstly, you will be killing two birds by one stone because if you complete HIIT Circuits a few times a week you will be burning fat as well as building/maintaining lean muscle mass – it's such an effective training method. Secondly, the list of benefits of having lean muscle mass is just brilliant. Just look at this list:

- Increased metabolism
- Increased hormonal stability.
- Increased longevity and vitality.
- Reduced risk of illness.

They are just some of the benefits. If you are planning to lose weight and not build any muscle mass, then you will just become skinny. You may think that being skinny is not a bad thing, but it is still unhealthy, unattractive and makes exercise harder to complete as your muscles may be too weak to create movement for a sustainable period.

HIIT Circuits that include explosive bursts of exercise (squat jumps are a good example of these bursts) may be more effective in boosting your V02 Max. V02 Max is the maximum consumption of oxygen measured during exercise, a high V02 Max is very beneficial to your health because it allows more oxygen and nutrients to get to your muscles meaning that your muscles will be able to perform at their best possible ability. Another benefit is that that you will be able to exercise at higher intensities for a longer time before becoming exhausted. Plus, you will be able to hold your breath for longer which can help with meditation and unexpected situations. Your body can use the oxygen more efficiently.

HIIT improves glucose metabolism. Metabolism is explained in the diet section of this book, but to put it simply. An improved glucose metabolism allows for the food you consume (Carbohydrates for this example) to be transferred into energy for your body more efficiently which will help your body and brain function better.

## Equipment

Don't worry, <u>not</u> one piece of equipment listed below is <u>needed</u> to complete any of the Circuits. The list of equipment below is all optional, the reason this is included is because each piece of equipment can be helpful towards your training routine.

- Skipping Rope – One of the exercises included in this book can be done with a skipping rope, but it can also be done if you are pretending to skip so it's not needed.

- Fitness Watch – A watch that will accurately measure your heart rate. This can be pricey but will help you manage to train in the correct training zone during exercise.

- Stopwatch – You will just need something to help you keep track of time while training, because it's easy to lose track of time which may mess up the Circuit.

- Fitness Mat – Helpful for when you are completing workouts on the floor, back in the day I used to work out on a towel laid out on the floor!

- Clothing – Just because you are at home doesn't mean you should exercise in your dressing gown. You should have the correct sports clothing when exercising because this will protect you from the environment – for example loose clothing is more likely to get caught on things and heat you up much more than shorts and a t-shirt/top would.

# Chapter 2 – The Diet for Effective Fat Burning

As a living being, it is probably a good idea that you eat food. Many people eat because of the feeling of hunger or because they crave a certain food that tastes nice. Although that is a good thing that people eat so that they avoid starvation, eating can become a bad habit because not all food is good for the body.

At the end of the day, food and drink is fuel for the body to keep it working. The body requires a good supply of six essential nutrients to function to the best of its ability. In the previous book "Intermediate Circuit Training" I went into much more detail about these nutrients, what they do, the sources of each nutrient and so on. To keep it short and sweet the six nutrients are:

- Water

- Vitamins

- Minerals

- Fats

- Carbohydrates

- Protein

## Energy

I hope that you have heard of each nutrient listed, if you haven't then you will be familiar with the essential nutrients shortly. Each of these nutrients play a large part in providing your body with energy. The nutrients are all found in food, drinks or supplements, so unless you starve yourself then you will be consuming these nutrients on the daily. It is unlikely that you will be severely lacking these nutrients from your current diet, although it is likely that you may not be getting enough of everything which can cause minor symptoms like a lack of energy, dry skin or an itchy scalp.

Your body needs energy for several reasons. The main reason is that your body uses the energy from food and drink to function. The body uses the energy form called ATP (adenosine triphosphate) and this is just like gas in the tank. This gas is used to maintain the body's essential functions like growth, repair, blood transport and it also fuels the muscles and the brain, which is essential to keep you functioning normally, exercising, thinking and so on...

For this book, the main reason for you need to get as much energy in your body as you can because it reflects on how you train. If you can't get enough energy because you don't eat enough, or you eat the wrong kind of foods, or your eating routine is too spaced out then your body will struggle to maintain a good energy level, which will end with you struggling to complete intense exercise.

Energy in food is usually measured by calories. Everyone is different and requires a different number of calories every day, calories are needed for metabolism, physical activity and other things that you may not pay much attention to. The general recommended daily calorie intake for men is 2500 and 2000 for women, as you will want to use every single calorie efficiently to reach your fitness goal then yours will be different. To discover your recommended calorie intake, then you will have to do some maths by following the formulas below:

Adult male: BMR = 10W + 6.25H - 5A + 5

Adult female: BMR = 10W + 6.25H - 5A − 161

W is body weight in kg

H is body height in cm

A is age

I find that a weird formula, but most importantly it allows for you to work out your Basal Metabolic Rate, you will learn more about this under the subchapter metabolism however for now you will need you BMR to insert into the formulas below. Please only select one of the options that applies to your current exercise situation.

1. If you are moderately active (moderate exercise/sports 3-5 days/week): Calorie-Calculation = BMR x 1.55

2. If you are very active (hard exercise/sports 6-7 days a week): Calorie-Calculation = BMR x 1.725

3. If you are extra active (very hard exercise/sports & physical job or 2x training): Calorie-Calculation = BMR x 1.9

Now you will have a number which is specific to you, this is the number of calories that you should aim to consume every day. This is the energy your body needs for functioning, for exercise and other things. You don't have to make sure you consume that exact number of calories each day, as long as it is close enough then it will help you burn fat, build lean muscle and provide your body with energy. If you exercise less than 3 times a week then that's what you should work towards before getting into HIIT Circuits!

## High Protein Diet

I would like to firstly clear something up, when I say you should try get as much energy as you can into your body – I do not want you to constantly stuff your face with snacks and treats, just because they may be high in carbs and provide plenty of energy doesn't mean it will be good for you.

Instead, you have to split up your diet. The reason why you want to split up where you get your energy from is because that not all energy sources are good for the body, some nutrients that provide energy may be good for you but once you have too much then that excess energy will be stored as excess fat.

As you are soon to be HIIT Circuit experts, I suggest you follow a high protein diet plan. The High Protein should be made up of around 40% of foods high in protein, 30% of foods high in fat and 30% of foods high in carbohydrates. Use calories as a system of measurement, I previously asked you to work out your recommended calorie intake and now you will have to split it up to meet these requirements. I say around 40% for foods high in protein because that should allow you to reach your recommended protein intake for if you are building muscle. Even if you do not want to build muscle - I still suggest a high protein intake because it plays an important role in your body and excess protein isn't harmful. Below you will find all the previous six essential nutrients which are all explained briefly on how they work and where they can be found (more information in previous books).

**40% Protein** – Foods that are high in protein basically make up this diet plan, so that's why just under half of your day will consist of eating foods high in protein. This may seem like too much protein, and for those of you who have low muscle mass then it is too much. Fortunately, too much protein doesn't do any harm apart from making your farts stink – yep that's true. So, make sure you have at least 40% of your daily diet covered by protein but the more you have is better and will keep your muscles strong.

Your body needs around 1.2g – 1.7g of protein per kilo of your body weight so that the muscles can grow and repair stronger after exercise, using myself as an example 80kg x 1.5 = 120 grams of protein every day. Unfortunately, consuming all this protein will not automatically make you look like Arnold Schwarzenegger – you will have to complete exercises consistently which cause the muscle to rip slightly so it can grow back stronger. Although I don't think you should worry about building muscle too much, if you stick to this diet and a training routine with HIIT Circuits I am sure you will have no trouble gaining lean muscle mass – if you are worried about gaining too much muscle mass the body weight exercises won't allow you to build too much!

Foods that are high in protein can be found here: Eggs, lean meats, poultry, salmon, beans, cheese, and natural peanut butter. With there being many more foods out there with similar protein properties. I also find protein shakes to be incredible protein providers. High protein foods are filling and make it harder for you to snack due to your filled stomach.

**30% Fats** – A decent chunk of the high protein diet should come from fat, this may sound stupid if this book is all about burning fat but let explain why this is the case. Firstly, you will find that some of the foods you consume that are high in protein are also reasonably high in fat – foods high in protein and fat will fill you up, will provide your body with enough energy and make it less likely for you to snack throughout the day.

There are good fats and bad fats, you will want to include both types into your diet but ideally consume more good fats than bad fats. The good fats are called: Polyunsaturated fats and Monounsaturated fats. While the bad fats are called: Saturated fats and Trans fats. You need to break up roughly how much of each you consume.

Out of the 30% for you daily fat intake, I would suggest for you to have 20% of that from the good fats and 10% from the bad fats.

Monounsaturated fats (good fats) are found in nuts, vegetable oils, peanut butter and avocados. While Polyunsaturated fats (good fats) are found in oily fish: Salmon, Herring, Trout, Sardines, and tuna, as well as tofu, walnuts, flaxseeds, vegetable oils and seeds. These good fats should make up roughly 20% of your daily diet, these will help reduce heart discase, lower the bad cholesterol and provide many health benefits.

Trans fats (bad fats) are found in fried food (doughnuts, fast-food), margarine, baked goods (cakes, pastries) and processed snack foods. You need to avoid Trans Fats because they provide no nutritional value and are damaging to the body – save these foods for the cheat day! Saturated Fats (bad fats) are found in high fat meats and dairy products such as: beef, pork, dark poultry, lamb lard, cheese, whole milk and tropical oils. 10% of your daily diet should come from Saturated Fats because your body needs fat for energy, and you will find it very hard to eat all that protein without consuming any saturated fat.

**30% Carbohydrates** – This diet plan requires a lower amount of carbohydrates than usually recommended, this may be a difference to your current diet because carbs usually make up a large part of our daily diet. Carbohydrates can be split into three types: sugar, starch and fiber. These carb types are either 'Simple carbs' or 'Complex carbs' because of how your body can deal with them for energy.

Simple carbs are easy to digest and are a good source of energy – natural simple carbs may be simple sugars found in fruit and added simple carbs are found in processed food or refined sugars like cake or sweets. Simple carbs are a good source of energy, but you have to stay away from the 'added sugars' because these are more likely to cause your blood sugar levels to spike which increases your appetite – "added sugar" carbohydrates are known as empty carbs because of they offer little nutritional value apart from a good taste. If you consume lots of foods high in protein then you will have an easy time cutting down the amount of simple carbs you have, I think Fruit and Lucozade are great sources of simple carbs that will help you get the energy you need.

Complex Carbohydrates take longer to be digested because they are formed in long complex chains. Complex carbs can be found in foods like wholemeal bread, wholemeal pasta, barley, quinoa, potatoes and corn. Complex carbs are rich in nutrients because they contain vitamins, minerals and fibre. Fiber is a brilliant nutrient because it fills you up, from the 30% of carbs that you will consume on the daily make sure to check the packing and look out for the foods highest in fiber because that sure will stop you snacking.

All carbohydrates are converted into glucose within the body, which is blood sugar, however depending on how easy they are to digest depends on how long it takes for the sugar to get into the blood. The simple carbs almost convert to glucose immediately, consuming a large amount of simple carbs is likely to increase your body fat percentage as the excess glucose that is not used by the body is converted to glycogen and is later stored as fat. Complex carbs provide your body with energy for a longer time period because of how long the take to digest, this is better for your body because it will keep you energised for longer and reduces snacking.

Complex carbs are a better source of energy for your body, but simple carbs from natural sources are also a good quick energy boost before a workout if needed. So, I suggest for you to have 5% of your daily calorie intake come from simple carbs such as fruit, milk or Lucozade's because these are the better options for simple carbs which contribute towards high energy levels. Please avoid the added sugars like cakes because they don't provide any sustainable energy. The other 25% should come from Complex Carbs, these will allow for you to maintain high energy levels throughout the day and reduce your appetite to reduce snacking.

**Vitamins** – Vitamins play a large part in the body as they perform hundreds of roles like bolstering your immune system and healing wounds. It is important you get a good supply of all the essential Vitamins like Vitamin A, Vitamin D, Vitamin K and so on. If you are sticking to this high protein diet, exercise regularly and go outside regularly then you won't fall short and should avoid the symptoms like having a lack of energy, or having poor vison. To be certain that you get all the essential vitamins you need to function to the best of your ability then I suggest taking Vitamin and Mineral tablets.

**Minerals** – Minerals are important because they keep your body functioning properly. Just like with vitamins, there is not really any reason to worry about consuming minerals as it is likely to be found in your food and drink. To ensure that you get all the minerals that you need (there are quite a few) then I would suggest taking vitamin and mineral tablets every morning.

**Water** – It is very important to stay hydrated. A good way to indicate whether you are hydrated is by looking at your pee, if your pee is transparent then you are hydrated, and your body would have flushed out the toxins and the water in your body can help transport nutrients around the body efficiently. However, if your pee is yellowish then that is a sign you are dehydrated and need to consume more water. Enough about pee, here are the facts you need. You should consume over 3 litres of water every day. Get into a routine of drinking water consistently throughout the day, don't try to drink 3 litres at once because that is extreme. Always have a glass/ bottle of water present when exercising because that is when your body needs water the most.

## Calorie Intake

This is an example of my calorie intake and how I would split it up every day between fats, carbs and protein. I am 180cm in height, 26 years old and 80kg in weight. So that means to work out my recommended calories I would do the following:

(10x80kg) + (6.25x180) − (5x26 years old) + 5 = 1800BMR.

I would then take that number then times it by 1.725 (I am very active, exercise 6-7 days a week) which means I would have to consume 3105 calories every day. That may be a lot, however I am very active with a muscle mass percentage higher than the average person, so keep that in mind.

Here is a website that you can use to measure your Calorie Intake which is much simpler than following that formula previously mentioned: https://www.calculator.net/calorie-calculator.html.

On this website you should be able to put in your info and click calculate to find your recommended calories intake, this will give you the same number as working out the formula. After that you will see a table with 4 different numbers on there, the highest number is your recommended calories which means if you consume that much following the high protein diet, they you will maintain your body weight (you will burn fat but build lean muscle mass as a weight replacement which is great).

Below your recommended calories you will see another 3 numbers which are lower than your recommended intake, for me those numbers are 2856 calories, 2606 calories and 2105 calories. By reading the chart you can see these are the calories you would have to consume to lose weight at a particular rate. I do not recommend following the bottom figure because there should be no need for you to lose weight at an extreme rate.

I suggest you either pick to eat your recommended calories for maintaining weight or to eat your recommended calories for mild weight loss. To continue using myself as an example, I will follow my recommended intake for mild intake which requires me to follow this formula:

(Recommended Calorie Intake for Maintaining Weight) x 0.92 = Recommended Mild Weight Loss Calorie Intake.

3105 Calories x 0.92 = 2856 Calories

Eating this number of calories will allow me to burn fat and lose a small amount of weight each week. At some point though you will have to eat the recommended amount to maintain weight because losing too much weight may not be what you are after. Below you can see how I can split up my day of eating to reach the 2856 calories.

40% of my daily diet will be made up of foods high in protein which means that I would consume roughly 1150 calories worth of lean meat, eggs, protein shakes, milk, beans, fish, cheese and other foods high in protein throughout the day. I make sure to have a large variety of proteins to make my day of eating enjoyable. Most importantly, I would make sure I meet my recommended protein intake for building muscle.

30% of my daily diet will consist of foods high in fat. More importantly 20% of the Good fats and 10% of saturated fat which would equivalate to around 300 calories of saturated fat and 600 calories from the Good Fats.

30% of calories come from Carbohydrates. To be more specific 5% will come from Simple carbs and 25% will come from Complex carbs. So roughly 100 calories worth of Simple but natural carbs and around 650 of calories from Complex carbs.

That is everything split up, it is now your turn to find out how many calories you require and how you are going to split it up. This is also a good place to address a cheat day, a cheat day is a day where you can enjoy all the foods you have been trying to resist because of how unhealthy they are. A cheat day once a week/two weeks is great because it gives you something to look forward to.

I don't need you to be exact with the calories you consume, as long you are within 50 calories for each requirement then your body will begin to make the positive changes. My day adds up to around 2800 calories which is good enough because remember you are still doing the exercise to help you get towards your goal.

## High Protein Diet Benefits

Below is a list of benefits of the High Protein Diet. I hope for this to prove why a high protein diet is the best option for those who want to burn fat quickly.

- Protein rich foods will reduce your appetite which will naturally prevent you from snacking and cravings. (Regular snacking is linked to putting on fat quickly)

- Protein is the building block of your muscles. A high amount of protein in your diet will allow you to build up lean muscle mass and become stronger as the circuits provide exercises that exert your muscles.

- Good for your bones as protein helps increase calcium absorption.

- Protein boosts metabolic rate by 20-35%, this will help your body burn calories more efficiently.

- Lowers blood pressure – a real good benefit to your overall health.

There are many other diet plans out there to help with fat burning, which I believe for the keto diet to be very popular at the moment. If you don't think the high protein diet will benefit you then feel free to follow a different diet plan that suits you. I understand some of you reading may be vegetarians or lactose intolerant which does restrict where you can get your protein from – although it doesn't make it impossible, so do your best to get all the protein you need.

**Foods to Avoid**

Straight to the point, below are foods and drinks that you should cut out from your diet. If you really struggle to resist the urge to eat these treats, then I am sure a cheat day once a blue moon won't hurt. Life is too short to constantly restrict yourself of these treats – as long as you make sure it is only once a blue moon.

- Foods and drinks high in sugar – like Coca Cola, Chocolate, Sweets, Cookies are all high in sugar. These treats will cause spikes in your blood sugar levels that cause hunger and as we know hungry people just keep eating and keep gaining weight. The excess glucose from the sugary foods is stored as glycogen in the liver – overtime this turns into fat which will make your belly look rounder.

- Alcoholic drinks – Wine, Beer, Spirits are all bad for you. Now if you enjoy a drink or two like me, then cut down on how often you have a drink and arrange for a night to drink once a blue moon (maybe on your cheat day?). Drinks that contain alcohol are not good for you because alcohol contains many toxins that are damaging to the liver, the heart and the effects of alcohol can damage your mental health over the long term. So, enjoy a glass every now and then, just don't drink consistently.

- Processed food (if you can) – Unfortunately, it is very difficult to go a day without eating something that is processed. Processed foods contain high amounts of added sugar, fat and sodium which isn't want our body wants in large quantities. Plus, I couldn't even begin to tell you all the ingredients they use for some processed foods, some of the stuff sounds like elements off the periodic table!

- Snacking – I understand that there is no food out there called "Snacking", but this is included because it is vital that you cut down on all the treats and snacks throughout the day. It is common to get the urge to enjoy a quick chocolate bar or cookie because it tastes nice and when you are bored eating helps pass the time. One snack a day which is healthy will do no harm - examples of healthy snacks include nuts, a handful of berries, natural Greek yogurt, or Apple slices with peanut butter.

- Fruit Juices – This often catches people out because fruit is healthy right? Well yes, but not fruit juice. Most fruit juices have lots of added sugar and one glass of apple juice can contain enough sugar that you need for a day. So, limit how often you have fruit juice or just drink fruit juice without added sugars.

## Good foods for your Brain

Your brain is what controls your thoughts, memory, speech, movement, the function of your organs and much more. So, it is important we get the brain what it needs right?

**Oily Fish** – Be sure to include oily fish into your diet as they include a high amount of fat, protein and omega 3. The unsaturated fats found in the fish lower the blood levels of beta-amyloid (this is a protein that forms in the brain and is damaging). Eating oily fish a few times a week can improve brain power and reduce the risk of Alzheimer's disease. Examples of oily fish: salmon, cod, tuna and pollack.

**Green Leafy Vegetables** – These vegetables are high in Vitamin K, lutein, folate and beta carotene which are all brain healthy nutrients. Examples of leafy green vegetables are kale, spinach, collards and broccoli – I would suggest including these on the side of a high protein meal because I can't imagine Kale being enjoyable on its own.

**Berries** – Berries are great for you but in low quantities because they are simple (although natural) carbs which will spike your blood sugar level. Let me get to the reason why they are great, simply because they are loaded with antioxidants. Antioxidants help protect the brain cells from damage which will keep your thinking sharp and knowledge maintained.

**Tea + Coffee** – Tea has caffeine and L-theanine while coffee contains caffeine. These drugs (legal drugs) are good for the brain because they promote central nervous system stimulation. This means that alertness and focus of the brain is increased over a short period of time. This is the important part, please limit your intake of caffeine because too much is dangerous. Having a cup of coffee late at night will keep you awake for a long while, which may mess up your sleeping pattern. I am sure that some of you enjoy a cup of coffee as soon as you wake up, which is great, stick to a cup a day and look out for the training tips section in the next paragraph to learn how caffeine can help you with exercise and fat burning.

Remember to take these into consideration with your diet plan, don't go constantly stuffing your face with oily fish because your body will lack the nutrients that the oily fish don't provide, it's all about splitting up your day of eating to meet the nutritional requirements. If your brain is healthy, then you will be healthy.

## Metabolism

Your metabolism is a term to describe all chemical reactions involved in maintaining the living state of the cells and organisms. The three main purposes of the metabolism are to: convert food to energy to run cellular processes, convert food to building blocks, and finally the metabolism has the purpose to eliminate metabolic waste. Overall, your metabolism is what converts food into energy.

Everybody has a different metabolic rate, the metabolic rate is the speed that the metabolism works at. Those of you who have a quick metabolic rate will be able to eat a lot without gaining weight because your body can burn more calories easily, while unfortunately those with a slow metabolic rate will find it easier to put on fat as not all the calories burn easily and the left-over calories store as fat. If you know you have a slow metabolic rate or you don't know your metabolic rate, it is still possible for you to burn fat, you will have to increase your metabolic rate. Before I get into that, you should know the categories of metabolism.

Basal Metabolic Rate (BMR) – This is your metabolic rate during sleep or deep rest. Your body is always working even at rest to make sure everything is functioning well, and this is the minimum calories needed to keep your lungs breathing, to control body temperature, to keep the heart beating and the brain fully functioning. Remember this is used to measure your daily calorie intake.

Resting Metabolic Rate (RMR): This is the lowest possible metabolic rate to keep your body functioning. This accounts for 50-75% of total calories used.

Thermic Effect on Food (TEF): This is the number of calories burned while your body digests food. This usually takes up around 10% of total calories used.

Thermic Effect of Exercise (TEE): Calories burned while exercising. This is something that will be high for all of you if you exercise HIIT regularly.

Non-Exercise Activity Thermogenesis (NEAT): This is the number calories required for simple activities such as standing, walking, fidgeting etc.

All the above contribute to how all the energy (calories) that you consume is being used every day. There are many contributing factors that affect your metabolic rate. A list of these is below, some of them are unable to be changed however I later suggest how you can make a change to these contributing factors to speed up your overall metabolic rate.

- Age – The older you are the lower your metabolic rate is. You are unable to go back in time unfortunately, however, don't let this put you off making an effort to increase metabolic rate, just see this as an obstacle if you are in that position.

- Muscle mass – The more muscular you are, the more calories you burn because your bigger muscles need more energy to maintain size and be used.

- Hormone disorders – Cushing's Syndrome and Hypothyroidism slow down your metabolic rate. For those that suffer with these disorders, don't let it stop you from training and increasing metabolic rate.

- Physical Activity – The more active you are, the more calories you burn. This factor can link to muscle mass as exercise allows for muscle mass to be increased.

- Temperature – When you are exposed to cold temperatures then your body needs to work harder and burn more calories to stay warm. But please don't feel the need to move to the artic, maybe just a cold shower everyday may help with this.

To help you lower your body fat percentage, lose weight or whatever your fitness goal is I suggest for you to try to increase your metabolic rate. This will allow you to burn more calories which will burn fat, will allow for you to maintain high levels of energy and below you can find a list of ways to increase metabolic rate which also contain their very own benefit to you mentally or physically.

- Consistent HIIT exercises – I mean this book alone covers all the benefits of HIIT Circuits and you will be able to try the HIIT Circuits included in this book to really see if they bring the positives mentioned.

- Consistent eating – By this I mean that you should space out your day of eating into 5 smaller meals to avoid going into starvation mode. Starvation mode is what your body goes into when you haven't eaten in a while and your body has to adapt to the lack of energy, which decreases your metabolic rate and also makes your body burn your muscles for energy, which lowers your muscle mass. So, avoid this starvation mode and eat regularly throughout the day to maintain a high metabolic rate. Don't stick to 3 meals a day!

- Eat lots of protein – This will be easy for you if you follow the high protein diet.

- Drink more water – Drinking water over sugary drinks is good for you because drinking at least 3 liters of water a day can increase metabolism by 10-30%.

- Drink Green Tea or Oolong Tea – These teas help convert some of your fat stored in your body into fatty free acid which increases fat burning by 10-17%.

- Eat Spicy Foods – Although I cannot take the heat, peppers contain capsaicin which can boost your metabolism. If you cannot handle the spice, then I understand if you avoid this because I can't handle it either.

All the methods above to increase your metabolic rate work differently for individuals, but if you want to get the best results you can then I suggest sticking to as many as them as you can – plus you will find yourself doing some of them naturally when in a fitness routine.

## When's the Right Time to Eat?

To be honest, there is not an exact answer to this question, but it is important you structure out your day of eating. Eating 5 or 6 smaller meals throughout the day is proven to provide many more benefits to your health and helps boost your metabolism compared to eating 3 meals a day. Try to leave around 3 hours between each meal, I will give an example of how to space out each meal:

1. Breakfast – Between 6am and 9am.

2. Mid-morning Meal – Between 9am and 12pm.
3. Lunch – Between 12pm and 3pm.
4. Mid-afternoon Meal – Between 3pm and 6pm.
5. Dinner – Between 6pm and 9pm.

Look at that! A great way to balance your day of eating out. If you like a healthy snack or two then feel free to snack between meals (if you are not training at that point) or before bed – just take into consideration the size of your snack.

Eating around a HIIT Circuit needs consideration. Eating too soon before or after a HIIT Circuit will most likely end with you vomiting because your body would not be able to digest food properly due to your high heart rate. I suggest that you consume a meal roughly 60 to 90 minutes before a HIIT Circuit, or you can consume a light snack around 30 minutes before if it fits into your eating routine. A pre workout meal or snack needs to be able to provide your body with enough energy to go ahead and complete the HIIT circuits. I feel slightly guilty for not providing many food examples in this book, so below is a list of light but healthy snacks/meals to enjoy roughly 30-90 minutes before a HIIT Circuit:

- Sliced banana on a rice cake.
- Greek yogurt with berries.
- Whole grain toast with nut butter or sliced meat.
- Oats with dried fruit.
- Hummus and pita bread.

It is a good idea to have a snack/meal after a HIIT circuit to replenish your body with nutrients and energy, this will also help with recovery. Here are a few meal ideas for 30 minutes after a HIIT session:

- Egg white omelet loaded with vegetables and a side of fruit.
- Peanut butter and banana in a whole grain wrap
- Oats with a banana and yogurt.
- A chicken or turkey sandwich wrap.
- Protein Shake with strawberries.
- Lean meats with quinoa and vegetables.
- Whole grain toast with peanut butter.

# Chapter 3 – How to Enhance Your Training

As you will be training at the top level, this chapter is dedicated to helping you exercise to the best of your ability to speed up progression towards your goal. You will find training tips to help you when it comes to exercise, goal setting techniques to refuel your ambition and plenty of other tips to contribute towards your goals.

## Rest and Recovery

Resting and recovering is needed after a workout, especially when it comes to High-Intensity-Interval-Training. Whether you are training HIIT 4 days a week or 7 days a week then it is important you do the best you can to rest, recover and prepare for your next circuit. That's the main reason you want to rest and recover because if you have got a HIIT Circuit to complete in 30 minutes, but you are still knackered and aching from the HIIT Circuit you completed yesterday, then you will struggle to keep the training up to standards. Not to mention that rest and recovery prevents injury.

Below you can find a few ways which help your body recover after training, I expect you to follow most of these tips because if you don't then you simply won't be able to reach your goal.

- Rest – It's in the title. After a circuit, it's good to relax to lower your heart rate and take the stress of your muscles. Sleep is a big part of rest; you need 8 hours of sleep every night so that you can wake up feeling fresh and energized for the next day of exercise.
- Cooldown – A cooldown needs to be performed straight after the circuit. The benefits of cooldowns are explained in

470

chapter 5. Just get into the habit of cooling down after exercise, if you don't then your body will have a hard time adapting to the sudden change in heart rate.

- Stay Hydrated – While you are exercising you should always have a bottle of water laying around because you will be sweating, and the lost water needs to be restored. Also have a glass of water after a workout because you may still be sweating for a short while afterwards and you need to replace the lost fluid.

- Eat your proteins – As you are likely to be following a high protein diet then this will be easy for you. Getting in protein will help rebuild your muscles that have been slightly damaged during the workout.

- Electrolytes – As you sweat you lose electrolytes which are things like potassium, sodium chloride, magnesium and calcium. A light snack like fruit or a sports drink like Lucozade after the workout will replenish your electrolytes. It is common for electrolyte loss to cause cramps which you will want to avoid.

- Have a Proper Rest Day – May be difficult for those who exercise 7 days a week, but eventually you will have to give your body one full day to relax. A gradual buildup of stress and tension from exercise over a long period of time can set you up for a long-term injury in the future. If you do plan to exercise 7 days a week, try to fit in a rest day once a fortnight. In other words, don't let your mindset make you overtrain.

- Get a Massage/Myofascial Release – These methods are ways to physically take stress away from any sore muscles. A massage improves circulation which allows you to relax and it helps the muscle recover. Myofascial release is like giving yourself a massage with a foam roller, you roll the foam roller over the muscles that ache, and it will help improve circulation within that muscle.

- Ice Bath – A very popular recovery technique. Getting in and out of an ice bath will cause a sudden change in temperature meaning that our blood vessels constrict and dilate repeatedly. This is meant to flush out waste products in tissues causing a quicker recovery.

The tips above will help you increase your recovery time and prevent injury. The quicker your recovery time then the less time it takes for your body to repair from the previous workout. Once you have a great recovery time you will be able to exercise HIIT every day without a problem, if you are looking to train twice a day using HIIT Circuits and Weight Training then feel free but you must consider the muscle groups you are using, don't go all out by completing exercise that only use your arm muscles because the excess tension on your arm muscles may cause injury.


## Progressive Overload

Progressive overload is a key factor to use when it comes to making gains – whether that is to gain muscle mass, improve endurance or burn fat. I have used progressive overload in all my circuit training books with the six-week plans to help you make progress. Unfortunately, you will not be able to find a six-week plan in this book as I believe you can use the structure from the last two books to make your own specific training plan.

Enough of six-week plans. Progressive overload is where you increase the workload of the circuit overtime by increasing or decreasing variables. I like to use the Jumping Jack example to explain progressive overload. If you have an overweight person and an athlete in the same room and told them to complete 20 jumping jacks in 30 seconds then the overweight person will struggle to complete it and the athlete will be able to do it easily, right?

As the overweight person may not be used to exercise and weighs more, that means their heart must pump faster to pump more blood around the body to the muscles due to the workload, meaning that he has a higher heart rate. As the athlete's body has adapted to exercise then their heart rate would be lower, this means they must increase their workload to match the overweight persons heart rate.

This means as you get fitter from exercising and eating well then you will have to increase your workload over time so that you can maintain your heart rate for every HIIT Circuit session, the ways to increase the workload of a HIIT Circuit include:

Increasing time spent for each exercise – Only increase this variable by a second or two at a time because working at a high intensity for too long is risky. But increasing this by a couple seconds will maintain your high heart rate for longer which ends up with more fat burned.

Decreasing your rest period – Yet again, only decrease this for seconds at a time because resting between High Intensity Exercises is vital for recovery. Having a shorter rest period will give your heart rate less time to slow down meaning the workload is increased.

Increasing Heart Rate – Quite obvious, but if you manage to exercise at a faster pace, that will cause your heart to beat faster meaning you are increasing the overall workload of the HIIT Circuit.

Using Equipment – This doesn't apply to the exercises in this book, but it is a great thing to know because if you start using weights for some of the exercises, then the resistance caused by the extra weight will force your muscle to work harder, which means your heart pumps faster.

It is up to you to know when to use progressive overload in your training routine. Making a small change every week to your circuits that increase the overall workload, will help you reach your goals. Without progressive overload you may find yourself at a stage where you are not burning fat as effectively as you were at the beginning, once you reach your goal and want to maintain that goal then progressive overload is not as important. But I suggest you slowly increase the overall workload of your HIIT Circuits over time, remember that the circuits I have included are all at different difficulties so keep that in mind.

## Injury

Injury is a setback. I am sure many of you that have been training for years have been injured in the past and you know how unfortunate it is. While training at a top level, it is more likely for you to get injured due to the intensity you will be training at, that's why it is vital I cover the best tips to avoid injury.

- Warmup before Circuits. This is hopefully screwed into your brain by now.
- Cooldown after Circuits – Again will be screwed into your brain.

- Don't train if you feel a slight pain – Training with a slight injury makes it worse.

- Don't work too hard for too long - Very important in this book. I advise you not to massively increase the length of time that you are exercising for as your body will find in hard to cope.

- Wear appropriate Clothing/footwear – Wearing normal clothing may cause you injury because the grip on your footwear may cause you to slip or your top may be too baggie and get caught on an object.

- Stay hydrated/eat correct foods.

- Allow time to recover after training.

- Develop the correct mindset – Chapter 8 is heavy on mindset for a good reason. Because those of you reading this may be excited to train HIIT and may go "Over the Top", by this I mean people are so motivated to reach their goal that they put in extra training on rest days and push their body to the complete max. Although I like the motivation, you should know training too often links to injury – much more is said in Chapter 8 and hopefully will help you find your balance of training.

- Complete Proper Form – I hope that after reading Chapter 7, you will have no issue with form. However, it's a good idea to practice exercises until you get it right before using them in a HIIT Circuit, because if you complete an exercise at a high intensity with the incorrect form that is likely to make you use your muscles out of balance – extra exercise on muscle groups because of balance issues may cause injury.

In Chapter 8 you can find plenty of information about an injury setback plan which is under the subchapter "More Motivation". To put it shortly a setback plan is a plan for how you will cope under the unfortunate circumstance of injury, this plan will help you turn a bad situation into a learning process and come back stronger than ever before.

In my previous books I have always covered how to prevent injury and it is hard for me to come up with new ideas to do with prevention as there is only so much you can do, but here you can find ways to deal with injuries. Whether the extent of your injury is small or large I am sure this may help. As injuries aren't always possible to avoid, below is a list of ways to treat injuries:

- Stick Ice on it – Cover an icepack with a towel and rest it on the part of your body which is injured. Applying a cold object to the injury will reduce inflammation and numb the pain.

- Rest – Every day should be a rest day unless you can exercise without using the injured part of your body (check with doctor).
- Ibuprofen – This is a painkiller that will reduce the pain and bring down swelling. Yet again I advise you to check with your doctor because I don't know your medical history and certainly don't have too many of these!

If it is a serious injury, leave it to your doctor because they will certainly be better at offering advice and will recommend how long to have off exercising. Although this chapter may sound obvious, there are still so many people that forget to do the basis and it costs them later on. So, don't let that be you!

## Training Tips

Not your average Joe can complete these circuits, meaning you can consider yourself a proper athlete if you consistently train HIIT Circuits. As an athlete, you will always have to be on top form because one day that you miss, because you "couldn't be bothered", can be the difference between success and failure. That may sound extreme for those of you who just have the goal to lower your body fat percentage, but you still must fully commit if you want your dream body. So, this leads me to suggest some training tips that will help you in the long run, each tip will be able to make a positive contribution towards helping you reach your fitness goal.

**Glucose Before a Workout** – When you are training as hard as you possible can, you will need as much energy as you can get. That leads me to suggest glucose. Glucose is a type of sugar (simple carbohydrate) found in many foods, although I suggest in the diet section to restrict the foods you consume that contain simple carbohydrates as the glucose that your body doesn't use is stored as fat, I suggest this for a pre workout meal/drink because you will be using up that glucose. As long as you get your glucose supply from something natural (no added sugar). A couple examples of having glucose before a HIIT Circuit include:

- Drinking a Lucozade 30 minutes before a HIIT Circuit.
- Having a handful of fruit 30 minutes before a HIIT circuit.

Glucose is a relatively healthy simple carbohydrate that can, as long as it is not consumed in large quantities, help you get the energy you need for the workout. Glycogen is stored after excess glucose is consumed, after a while that glycogen is turned into fat which will increase body fat percentage (specifically around the belly area). Muscles use glycogen for energy, so that is why when you need this for a workout.

**Caffeine Before a Workout** - Secondly, I suggest for you to drink a caffeinated drink like coffee or an energy drink around an hour before a workout. This is because caffeine increases the brains alertness and arousal levels which tricks the brain to think the workout is easier than it actually is. Caffeine gives your body a big energy boost around 15 to 60 minutes after consumption which will help your body cope to the training load. What I find best about a pre workout caffeinated drink is that caffeine can shift muscles to burn fat quicker, preserve the glycogen store and allow for the muscles to work for longer and harder before wearing out. A drink that contains roughly 100mg of caffeine will do the job, obviously if you don't like caffeinated drinks or your body has a bad reaction to caffeine, then avoid them.

**Extra Salt** – Please take this with caution. As HIIT Circuits are difficult it will make you sweat more and lose more fluid. Salt (sodium chloride) is lost throughout the day because it leaves the body through sweat and urine – meaning for those that drink lots of water and exercise hard, you will need more salt in their body. It is impossible for me to suggest how much salt for you to consume daily because everyone's body is different, the recommended amount of salt is less than 6 grams a day. I suggest for you to consume between 5 to 6 grams of salt a day. Cramps usually occur when you do not have enough salt and it is common to have more cramps when consistently training at a higher intensity. So, get all the salt you need to stop them cramps causing you trouble.

**The Wim Hof Breathing Technique** – I am always researching ways in which can be beneficial to help people reach their fitness goals. I came across this guy on YouTube, Wim Hof, he has his own breathing technique that helps him with all sorts of extreme things – this man once ran a marathon in a desert with no water! The idea of his breathing technique is for the lungs to intake more oxygen than is released over a certain period which makes your blood more alkaline and causes hypoxia. This breathing technique could be considered as meditation and comes with many benefits.

This breathing method has been tested by scientists for many years now on normal people, like yourself, to prove that Wim is not a superhuman and the results show that it can bring a few benefits such as: increased energy, better sleep, increased determination, improved sports performance, stronger immune system, faster recovery and greater cold tolerance to anyone that consistently uses the breathing technique.

The breathing technique consists of 30 quick deep breaths (in through your nose and out through your mouth), followed by a large inhale and exhale to which you will then hold your breath for as long as you can before having to inhale, after the final inhale you hold your breath for 15 seconds. You can repeat this method up to 3 times. I strongly suggest giving this a try and follow his guided breathing technique on YouTube as that makes it easier to follow. From personal experience, I can say this method helps relax me which is a positive because I find myself to be restless in the evening – relaxation is important for recovery and growth.

I don't want to take any credit from the main man Wim Hof, that's why if you are interested, I suggest you check out his YouTube video on how to follow the Breathing Technique and find out all the benefits that come with it. Just to point out, this isn't something that will change your life overnight but if you stick to 10 minutes a day of mediation, eventually you will notice the positive changes it makes to your life.

https://www.youtube.com/watch?v=tybOi4hjZFQ

**Stretching** – Although you will stretch before and after each HIIT Circuit or workout, I still suggest for you to stretch regularly. An example of stretching regularly is waking up every day and starting your day with 10 to 15 minutes of deep stretches to extend your range of motion. The benefits of regular stretching can be found in the list below. Before I get to the list, this is a good opportunity for those with slight injuries or knocks such as back pain, stiff joints or sprained ankles to relieve all that stress put on their body and get prepared for exercise. The benefits include:

- Increases Flexibility — crucial for overall health and helps with everyday activities.
- Increases range of motion — this will give you more freedom of movement.
- Increases blood flow to muscles — this will shorten your recovery time and reduces muscle soreness.
- Great for Stress Relief — when you experience emotional or physical stress then your muscles are tense, meaning regular stretching will reduce stress held in places like your neck, shoulders and upper back.
- Improves posture — good posture brings a number of benefits, the most common one being that it will reduce back pain.

Now, it is probably a good idea that you put this to the test although that can be quite hard if you don't know what stretches to do, not to worry because I include a few stretches that you can try out every day.

**Standing Hamstring Stretch** – Stretches your hamstrings. 1) Stand with feet slightly apart and knees slightly bent. 2) Slowly bend your body forwards at the hips and lower your head towards the floor. 3) Reach down as far as possible with your arms to feel the stretch in your hamstrings and hold that position for 30 seconds before slowly standing back up.

**Seated Shoulder Squeeze** – Stretches your deltoids and great for fixing posture. 1) Sit on the floor with knees bent and feet flat on the floor. 2) Take your arms behind your lower back and lock fingers. 3) Straighten and extend your arms to squeeze your shoulder blades together. Hold that for 3 seconds and continue to repeat that a few times.

**Knee to Chest Stretch** – Stretches your lower back and glutes. 1) Lay down on the floor facing the ceiling/sky and use your arms to hold your knees into your chest. 2) Keep your lower back on the floor and apply extra force to push your knees into your chest to feel the stretch – hold for 30 seconds.

**Extended Puppy Pose** – A great stretch for your back. 1) Start on your hands and knees but have your arms fully extended in front of you, keeping your palms planted to the floor. 2) Push your hips up and back towards your heels. 3) Push through your palms onto the floor and you should feel the stretch across your back and shoulders – hold for 30 seconds.

**Butterfly Stretch** – Great stretch for Hips. 1) Sit on the floor with a straight back, knees bent out to the side and soles of feet together. 2) Hold your ankles, engage your core and slowly lower your chest towards your feet. Also press your knees towards the floor, hold this stretch when you can feel it in your legs and back for 30 seconds. 3) Once stretched, slowly raise your body back to the starting position and repeat a couple times.

**Seated Neck Release** – Great stretch to relieve tension from your neck. 1) Sit with your back straight and chest lifted. 2) Roll your neck to the left so your left ear almost touches your left shoulder. 3) You can press down gently on your head to extend the stretch and hold this for 30 seconds before repeating on the right side.

There you have it, just a few of these stretches which will take up 10 minutes of your day will help you gain all the benefits previously listed. You can also use the stretches included in the warmups to help improve flexibility. Please check out this website to find more detailed explanations and picture examples for each stretch.

https://www.self.com/gallery/essential-stretches-slideshow

## Finding Time

Many of us have busy lives, to which may make it hard for you to find time to complete these HIIT Circuits. Although one HIIT circuit will take up roughly 20-30 minutes of your time, it still can be hard to find this time for when you are tired, working, looking after somebody or whatever else it may be. Unfortunately, I am not going to let that from stopping you get your workout in.

Break your day up, everyone has 24 hours in a day, but some people manage to get so much more done that others in the same time period, Kevin Hart or Joe Rogan are great examples of people who manage this. You need 8 hours to sleep, which leaves roughly 16 hours for you to do all your day-to-day activities. It sounds like lots of time, but it can go quickly and before you even know it you have missed your workout and you are behind on your work. Fortunately for you, I have included a list of tips to help you increase your productivity:

Don't snooze – Before you go to bed set your alarm in a place where you will have to physically get out of bed to turn it off, because once you are up you will not be tempted to go back to sleep. Once you are up, you will have a fresh and longer day to look forward to because you have added 9, or 18, or 27 minutes to your day by getting up earlier than usual.

No daytime TV – First of all, what is on TV during the day that is worth watching? Because I don't think there is anything decent on TV until the evening, if you do like a certain program that's on during the day then just record it and watch it later. Use your day wisely to get things done and use the time to watch TV later in the day as a reward for getting it done.

Put your phone away – By this I don't mean for you to never touch your phone again, just put it away at times where you have stuff to do because it is a big distraction. For example, if you have an hour to get some work done, but you spend 20 minutes of that time scrolling on your phone then you have wasted 20 valuable minutes of work time, which will make you fall behind. It may be hard to concentrate for that entire hour, but once you hide the distractions like a phone, then you will find it much easier to crack out a solid hour of work and you may surprise yourself on how much you can get done.

Work when you work, rest when you rest – It's no-good dedicating the next hour of your day towards getting some work done if you are actually just going to spend 10 minutes on your phone, 10 minutes eating, 5 minutes watching videos and so on. You must stick to it, if you can get that solid hour of work done then you will free up more time for later in the day where you can kick your feet up and enjoy your rest – more importantly this will open up time for you to exercise!

Meal Prep – Cooking can take a while sometimes and leave you frustrated as you know you can use that time to do other things. That's why cooking in bulk for a few days will save you time later on in the week when you need it, as long as you have containers and space in your fridge you can cook meals for the future – just make sure to not prepare for too far in the future as food can go off!

Following these tips above should allow you to free up your time during the day, just freeing up a solid 30 minutes will allow you to get a great workout in. There is no better feeling than getting everything done in a day.

## Goal Setting

You need a goal. Why you ask? Well because having a set goal gives you something to work towards and is a way for you to track your progress. You will need to set yourself smart goals. A smart goal should be:

**Specific** – This means for the goal to suit you. If you want to lower your body fat to 5% then write it down!

**Measurable** – This means that you can track your progress towards your goals. A goal to lower body fat is perfect because you can use Skinfold Calipers to measure your current body fat percentage to see if you are on target.

**Attainable** – The goals must be possible. If you set a goal that is way of out of reach within that time limit, then you may be putting lots of unwanted pressure on yourself to perform. This can lead to stress and disappointment for when you fall short of your goals.

**Relevant** – It must make sense. If you are looking to lower your body fat percentage, setting a goal to snap a pen in half makes absolutely no sense. Although I have taken that wrong example to an extreme, it still applies. Instead, your goal should be to lower your body fat percentage to 5%.

**Time-bound** – Your goals need a time limit towards it. Without a time-limit then it is less likely that you will reach your goals because there is no urgency for you to complete the goal.

The reason I say that you need to set Smart Goals, and not just a smart goal is because you should be setting 3 smart goals. They should be short-term, medium-term and long term. This puts you in a position where you will always have a goal to work towards, and once you reach your long-term goal then you will have to set another short-term, medium-term and long-term goal (even if that is to maintain your current body fat percentage) because that will keep you in a healthy routine. A short-term goal should have a time limit between a month and 3 months, medium term goal should be between 3 and 6 months while finally a long-term goal should be 9 months to a year.

If you don't know how to make your goals specific then think about what you want, if you want to look more toned/defined then your goal should be based on lowering body fat percentage (use skinfold calipers to measure progress). If your goal is based on looking bigger then focus on building lean muscle mass. If you goal is to become fitter over short distance events like sprinting, swimming or so on then use HIIT to increase your anaerobic endurance. Whatever your goal may be, simplify it and use the internet to search how you can measure your muscle mass, anaerobic capacity or whatever it may be.

# Chapter 4 – How to Train Towards Completing HICT

When people have a goal of running a marathon, they don't just try to run it without any training because that is not the best idea. Unless you are God himself, then there is not a chance that you will be able to finish the marathon without training for it, because you have not given your body enough time to adapt to it. The same goes for HIIT Circuits. If you haven't exercised in a few months and you think that you will be able to complete a HIIT Circuit with no problem, then think again. I do not want to stop people trying a HIIT Circuit because they are too unfit to complete it, although yes, I understand that I have said this book is not for the beginners, they can still give It a go and train towards completing a HIIT Circuit.

Like I have repeated too many times throughout this book, I do not know the ability of everyone that is reading. So, if you don't know whether you can complete a HIIT Circuit or not, then try to complete the first HIIT Circuit in Chapter 6 and see how it goes. If you had to stop after a minute then no worries, you made a good attempt and I suggest looking at the previous books of this series so that you can get into a routine. If you completed over 50% of the circuit then well done, this book is good for you and you will be able to work towards completing it one day. If you managed to complete it relatively easily, then I suggest skipping this chapter – although that is quite stupid of me to say because the Circuits are in Chapter 6 and people don't usually read a book back to front... Anyway, maybe its best you refer back to this chapter after reading this book and completing a circuit.

## Record

If you are at a stage where you can't complete the entire circuit, but you're not far off, then please don't give up because I am here to help you. After attempting a HIIT circuit it is important that you record what you have done. There are many things to record as there are many variables but below are the important variables to help you make progress.

Record the heart rate you were working at during the circuit. See if it was similar to the required Heart Rate listed on the Circuit. Record how long that you were exercising in the HIIT Circuit before having to stop to catch a breath. Finally, record any other things that happened while you were completing the circuit – if you needed a longer rest between exercises then note it down and so on.

Now that you have noted everything down, you will easily be able to see how far away you are from completing a HIIT Circuit. It is now up to you to set goals to improve certain aspects of your HIIT Circuit.

Example: For my first try at a HIIT Circuit I managed to follow the requirements for 10 minutes before having to come to a stop because I was out of breath. For the next time I train I want to try completing another 20 seconds of the HIIT Circuit before coming to a stop. I will continue to do this until I can fully complete the circuit. However, if I am able to complete another 20 seconds each HIIT Circuit session without being completely out of breath I will train for a bit longer until I have to stop.

**Take-Action**

Now it's your turn to take-action. The last subchapter suggests you record your results of the HIIT Circuit that you completed as a 'Test'. From those results you should be able to see a clear goal you have set yourself and it is now your turn to work towards them. Sticking with the previous example, you should complete the warmup then set up a timer for 10 minutes 20 seconds for when you next train the HIIT Circuit and aim to train until the timer finishes – you can even choose to carry on exercising for longer if you feel up to it. It is now your job to track your progress, so if you have trained an extra 30 seconds than the previous session, then note that down so you can aim to train for another 20 seconds past your personal best. Eventually, you will be at a stage where your goal to add an extra 20 seconds to each session will mean that you would have completed the entire HIIT circuit.

Unfortunately, taking action is easier said than done – but that doesn't mean it is not possible. You will need to self-motivate yourself to pick yourself up and train harder in each HIIT Circuit until you get to a stage where you can complete a HIIT Circuit from start to finish. It is more of a mental game from this point, the last Chapter in this book titled "Improvise, Adapt and Overcome" you will find plenty of motivational tips, advice on how to develop a determined mindset which will help you reach any goal you set yourself.

## Improve

Progress is almost guaranteed to happen if you stick to a plan. The plan that includes a healthy diet and a consistent training routine with progressive overload will certainly let you improve to a stage where you can complete a HIIT Circuit. This is the fun part, where you can record your progress and feel proud of what you have achieved. Use your progress information to see if your goal can be achieved in a quicker period.

I suppose that you will be able to complete the HIIT Circuit after a while, and when you get to that stage, congratulations. You have reached your goal, but it shouldn't stop there. You should now introduce a variety of HIIT Circuits into your training routine, set yourself the 3 smart goals and keep pushing to improve. If you get to a stage where you feel you cannot set new goals as you don't feel the need to, then your goal should be to maintain your progress. Without maintaining, you will get back to a stage where you become unhealthy and struggle to complete a circuit.

**Are you a Beginner?**

I may have mentioned many times that this book isn't suitable for beginners, but if you are a beginner and want to give it a go, I am not going to stop you. This sub-chapter is just for any people who may be in a position where they haven't exercised for months, they don't know much about a healthy diet or a good exercise routine and the basics of keeping fit. It is completely fine if you are in this position because we all have to learn somehow.

People that get started with exercise are more likely to get injured because they don't know what they are doing, they try to rush things, or they have restrictions holding them back. Any restrictions like back pain, pain/stiffness in your joints, sprained ankles and so on all make the likelihood of you getting injured during exercising quite high, these restrictions can be formed over a lifetime. Luckily, these restrictions can be reversed with a number of methods so hopefully make exercising less painful and worthwhile for you in the future. In "Circuit Training for Beginners" you can find many gentle stretches, exercises and a recovery plan which will prepare your body slowly so you can start exercising safely.

Starting something new is always tough, especially when the workload is much higher than recommended. But don't let that discourage you, I am always here to support you. What to take from this: if you are a beginner then I suggest getting into a light exercise routine before tackling any of the HIIT Circuits. Slow and steady wins the race, so use the advice given in this chapter to work towards completing a HIIT Circuit.

# Chapter 5 – The Warmups and Cooldowns for HICT

A very straight forward chapter that contains warmups and a cooldown. You should know how important it is to prepare for a workout by warming up beforehand, I am sure most people know this but either can't be bothered to do so or forget about it. It is also important to cool down after a workout, people are more likely to forget the cool down because they think they have completed the workout and want to get on with the rest of their day.

## Warmups

Warmups are essential to carry out before training, the idea is to raise your heart rate and loosen the muscles you will use in the workout. You will need to raise your heart rate to around 70% to 80% of your max heart rate during the warmup to prepare for HIIT, this is so the right nutrients and oxygen is delivered to the muscles so they can perform at a high intensity. Without a warmup, it is highly likely you will suffer an injury.

Below you can find the heart raisers and stretches that make up "Warmup 3" and "Warmup 4". It comes clears that in this series the warmups and cooldowns are linked to the circuits later provided in this book. So, make sure you have a good look at the HIIT Circuits to see how they match up with the warmups, the harder HIIT Circuits are more likely to link to Warmup 4.

Warmup 3 (5 Minutes) –

- Light Jog on Spot – 1 minute
- Walking Knee Hugs – 30 seconds
- Sexy Circles – 30 seconds

- Arm Extension Hold – 30 seconds
- Ankle Rolls – 30 seconds
- Lateral Split Squat Stretch – 30 seconds
- High Kick Outs – 30 seconds
- Heel Flicks – 1 minute

Warmup 4 (5 Minutes)

- Light Jog – 1 minute
- Childs Pose – 30 seconds
- Calves Stretch – 30 seconds
- Hamstring Stretch – 30 seconds
- Chest Stretch – 30 seconds
- Side Lunge – 30 seconds
- Backpedaling – 30 seconds
- 5 Burpees (Do this in your own time)

## Cooldowns

As explained before, cooldowns take place after a workout to allow gradual recovery by lowering the heart rate slowly. Stretches are certainly needed after a HIIT circuit as your muscles would be tighter after a high intensity session. Cooldowns should be slow, while including a range of stretches to increase the range of motion and light exercises to bring down the heart rate. Cooldowns typically last around 3 to 5 minutes. I will list a good cooldown to perform after a HIIT circuit:

Cooldown 3 (5 minutes)

- Light Jog on Spot – 60 seconds
- Lunges – 30 seconds
- Close the Gates – 30 seconds
- Seated Spinal Twists – 30 seconds
- Neck Rolls – 30 seconds
- Calf Raises – 30 seconds
- Bicep Stretch – 30 seconds
- Shake off Arms and Legs – 60 seconds

There is a reason why these are included in this book, that's because you will do a warmup before every HIIT Circuit and a Cooldown after every HIIT circuit. You cannot create shortcuts, if you think these aren't important then please don't complain when you get injured because the most common injuries are caused by skipping the warmup and cooldown. Although I may be sounding harsh, people don't always follow the basics and its costs them, I have always loved to take shortcuts, but it eventually caught up with me. Moral of the story: Don't cut corners!

# Chapter 6 – The High Intensity Circuits to Burn Your Body Fat!

Here are the tough circuits I bet you cannot wait to smash through. There are five HIIT circuits that go up in difficulty. The five main circuits are titled "HIIT Circuit 1", "HIIT Circuit 2", "HIIT Circuit 3", "VHIIT" and "100%". Just like normal, all circuits are listed with all the exercises, the warm-ups and the cooldowns that link to them. You can find the warmup and cooldowns in Chapter 5 as well as find the exercise descriptions in Chapter 7.

As previously explained, HIIT stands for High Intensity Interval Training and VHIIT stands for Very High Intensity Interval Training – this should give the message that not everyone will be able to complete the circuits like planned. Although that doesn't mean you cannot have a go at them, just work to the requirements that are located above the circuit and do your best. If you came from the previous book and gave the HIIT taster a good go then you should be ready to include more HIIT circuits into your fitness routine.

I have tried my best to include a range of exercises for each HIIT Circuit so that you are working most muscle groups in the body – a whole body workout also provides great balance and won't leave you looking top heavy! Also check out the Abdominals HIIT Circuit, this is specific to training your core which helps burn belly fat.

## What Makes HIIT Circuits Harder?

This short segment will provide you with enough information to make your own circuits. A standard circuit that you can find in my other two books and it is very similar to a HIIT circuit because it contains a list of exercises with a period of rest in-between. The main difference between HIIT Circuits and Normal Circuits is that the rest period of the normal circuits is equal to the time spent exercising the exercise while the rest period is either slightly longer, equal or shorter in HIIT circuits – this is because rest is much more appreciated after working at a high intensity, so starting off with a longer rest makes the HIIT Circuit easier and the rest time can be reduced to pose a real challenge. The main difference is the increased intensity, you will discover how tough it is to exercise above 80% of your max heart rate, with the normal circuits you would have been working at an intensity below 80% which is easier for your body to recover from.

## HIIT Circuit 1

The first HIIT circuit of the book so that makes it the least challenging, although don't underestimate this circuit as it will still leave you sweating. This is the least difficult because it is the shortest to complete a set.

Complete 3 sets, Train in the Hard Training Zone (Around 80% of Max HR). Rest for 30 seconds between each exercise and rest for 2 minutes between sets. This circuit will take roughly take 25 minutes to complete including the warmup and cooldown.

Warmup 3

1. Burpees – 20 seconds
2. Bicycle Crunch – 20 seconds
3. Tuck Ups – 20 seconds
4. Shoulder Pushups – 20 seconds
5. Forward Kick Outs – 20 seconds

6. Open and Close Gates – 20 seconds

Cooldown 3

## HIIT Circuit 2

Complete 2 sets, Train in the Hard Training Zone (Around 80% of Max HR). Rest for 30 seconds between each exercise and rest for 2 minutes between sets. This circuit will take just over 25 minutes to complete including the warmup and cooldown. This circuit includes more exercises to increase the variety of the circuit, I have also alternated the time spent on each exercise to increase the difficulty.

Warmup 3
1. Lying Superman Hold – 30 seconds
2. Fast Feet – 15 seconds
3. Wall sit – 30 seconds
4. Twist and Point – 15 seconds

5.  Skipping – 30 seconds

6.  Flutter Kicks – 15 seconds

7.  Plank to Pushups – 30 seconds

8.  Side Plank – 15 seconds a side

Cooldown 3


## HIIT Circuit 3

Complete 2 sets, Train in the Hard Training Zone (Around 85% of Max HR). Rest for 20 seconds between each exercise and rest for 2 minutes between sets. This circuit will take just over 20 minutes to complete including the warmup and cooldown. Although this is shorter than the previous circuits, you are required to work hard.


Warmup 4

1.  Twist and Point – 20 seconds

2.  Snake Pushups – 20 seconds

3.  Mountain Climbers – 20 seconds

4. Squat Jumps – 20 seconds

5. Standing Side Crunches – 20 seconds

6. Ali Shuffle – 20 seconds

7. Straight Punches – 20 seconds

8. Lunges and Twist – 20 seconds

9. Wall Sit – Hold 20 seconds

10. Twist Jumps – 20 seconds

Cooldown 3


## VHIIT Circuit

Now it's time to move to the Maximum Training Zone, where the real gains are made. Your body may have not worked this hard in a very long time and to be honest, that's understandable.

Complete 3 sets, Train in the Maximum Training Zone (90% of Max HR). Rest for 30 seconds between each station and rest for 2 minutes between sets. This Circuit will take roughly 25 minutes to complete including the warmup and cooldown. Make sure to rest properly in the rest periods as you need all the energy you can get.

Warmup 4

1. Half Squat Jumps – 20 seconds
2. Power star – 20 seconds
3. Bicycle Crunches – 20 seconds
4. Mountain Climber – 20 seconds
5. Boxer Squats – 20 seconds
6. Fast High Knees – 30 seconds

Cooldown 3

## 100%

This one is mental, working at 100% of your heart rate is very hard to achieve but of course it is possible. As you are exercising as hard as you possibly can, the time spent on exercise will be short, but I will keep the rest periods short, so your heart rate doesn't drop dramatically.

Complete 2 sets, Train in the Maximum Training Zone (Work as hard as you can – 100% of Max HR). Rest for 20 seconds between exercises and 2 minutes between sets. Will take 20 minutes to complete including the warmup and cooldown. Do not attempt as a complete beginner. On your rests, I suggest sitting/standing upright with your hand behind your head to intake as much oxygen as possible.

Warmup 4

1. Fast Feet - 20 seconds
2. Burpees with Pushup – 20 seconds
3. Diamond Pushups - 20 seconds
4. Side Plank – 20 seconds
5. Reverse Crunches - 20 seconds
6. Squat Thrust – 20 seconds
7. Snake Pushups – As many as possible

Cooldown 3

If you are an absolute animal then you can make that circuit harder by adding more exercises, spending longer on each exercise. I managed to complete this circuit, but I was out of breath for ages afterwards. Feel free to share you experience within the Facebook group!

## Abdominal HIIT Circuit

I had to throw this in, it was only right because everyone wants a nice, toned stomach or six-pack. This circuit targets your abdominals and obliques to help you look great in front of a mirror with a strong core. From my experience, I find that abdominal workouts where there is little rest between the exercises allow for better results because the gains are made while the core is engaged – this is the reason for the short rests.

Complete 3 sets, Train in the hard training zone (Around 80% of Max Heart Rate). Rest for 10 seconds between each exercise and 2 minutes between each set. This will take you roughly under 20 minutes to complete including the warmup and cooldown.

Warmup 3

1. Bicycle Crunch – 20 seconds
2. Flutter Kicks – 20 seconds
3. Mountain Climber – 20 seconds
4. Plank to Pushups – 20 seconds
5. Knees to Chest – 20 seconds
6. Side plank – 20 seconds each side

Cooldown 3

I have managed to complete all these circuits, although I do admit the 100% circuit is ridiculous, it is still possible. Don't forget that I have been training for years and if you can't complete it the first time don't give up because it takes mental strength to complete, you will have to work towards it and enjoy doing so. The resistant exercises like push-ups or squats may make you feel like you are working slower compared to completing the other exercises, don't worry about this because your body has a harder time when having to push/pull bodyweight which will maintain your high heart rate even when you think you are training slowly.

## How Often to Train

If you have come from either of the previous two books, then you know that the recommended time for exercise is either 150 minutes of moderate physical activity or 75 minutes of vigorous activity.

You are now at a level where you should be way above the recommended time for exercise each week. I would suggest for those training at the top level to be training HIIT Circuits 6 or 7 days a week. For those working their way up towards completing a HIIT Circuit then I suggest training 4 days a week from the start and keep building up your workload until you reach 6 days a week. You can of course complete 3 days of HIIT and 4 days of weight training if you are looking to build up muscle quickly. There are so many ways you can include HIIT Circuits into your routine.

## Make Your own HIIT Circuit

Below I will give you a template of how you can create your own circuit. I think it is important to give people the option to train the way that suits them. Feel free to use the exercises included from any of the books in this series, or any of your own exercises that you love. Most importantly, make it fun. Below is the list of variables that you must fill in to make up the Circuit.

Number of Sets:

Training Zone:

Rest Time Between Exercises:

Rest Time Between Sets:

Time of Complete Circuit:

Exercises Included:

1.

2.

3.

4.

# Chapter 7 – Each Exercise With a Detailed Description and Photo

**HIIT 1 Exercises**

**Burpee** - Now this is a hard exercise to start with, but it is worth it. Start in the usual starting position. Then drop to the ground into a crouch position shown in the 1st photo with your hands planted on the ground. From the crouch position, stretch your legs out to a high plank position shown in the 2nd photo. Then you will want to hop your feet back into the first crouch position followed by a powerful jump upwards by pushing through your heels and hold your arms up to land like the 3rd photo shows (while in mid-air). You will then repeat all the above without resting for the time required. I recommend practising this exercise as you will

530

want to be quick with this in the HIIT Circuits. Burpees are a whole-body workout meaning they build muscular strength and endurance in the upper and lower body.

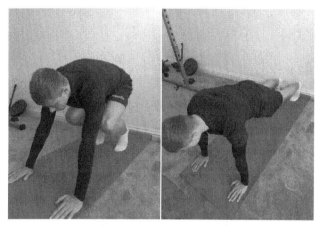

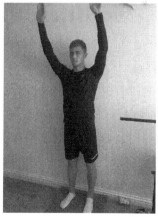

**Bicycle Crunches** - Lay flat on the floor facing the ceiling with both hands behind your head. Keep your head and shoulders lifted off the ground for the entire activity by using your arms to slightly pull away from the floor. Start by bending your left knee towards your chest while your right leg is bent with your right foot on the floor, while you bend your left knee to your chest, twist your upper body and head to the left and you should feel it in your obliques (side abs). From that position, extend your left leg out forwards, twist your body from left to right using your lower back and bend your right knee towards your chest. Continue to swap legs and twist from left to right, right to left for the time provided. This exercise is best for burning fat around the abdominal area, while working the rectus abdominals, hips and obliques.

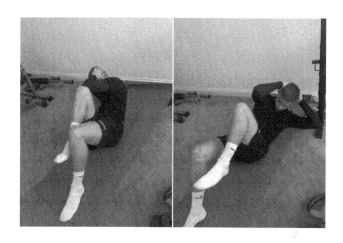

**Knees to Chest** – Lay on the floor facing the sky, with your legs fully extended. In one movement, bring your knees to your chest using your lower back and legs. Hold your legs in position (Photo 2) for a split second before relaxing your arms and pushing your legs back into the starting position (Photo 1). Continue to crunch your knees to and from your chest, this exercise is great for strengthening and defining your lower abs.

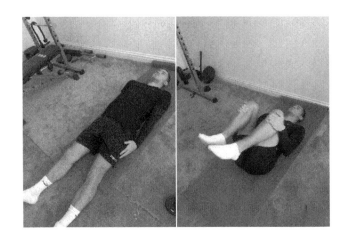

**Shoulder Push-ups** – Get into the position that the 1st photo shows, to do this plant hands on the floor so that they are in line with your shoulders, then place your tiptoes on the floor but stick your bum up and close the distance between your hands and feet. To do a shoulder push-up, keep your hands and toes planted and use your arms to lower your face near the ground, once you reach a stage where you can't go down any further push back using your arms. This mainly works your deltoids, making you work your shoulders as well as working chest and triceps.

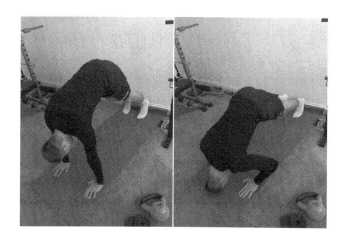

**Forward Kick Outs** – Stand on the spot keeping on your toes. Then simply just raise your left knee while keeping it bent (Kung-Fu Stance photo 1), after it is lifted maintain balance and in one motion you should kick out your left lower leg and bring it back in to the "Kung-Fu" stance. Lower your left foot to the ground and repeat with your right leg. This may not be the most intense exercise, but it improves balance, and it can be done quickly so that you will feel the burn at the end of a circuit.

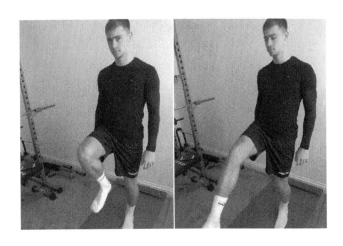

**Open and Close the gates** – A relatively gentle exercise for HIIT. Begin by standing up straight with your feet moderately apart, then lift your left knee up in front of you, move your leg roughly 90 degrees to the left by rotating your hip (keep foot off the ground). Now that you have opened the gate, you need to close the gate, do this by moving your left knee 90 degrees right then lowering your foot to the ground (Just reverse your movements from opening the gate). Repeat that on your right leg but rotate to the right instead of left when opening the gate. Great exercise for improving balance it also will work glutes, hamstrings and keep your hips loose.

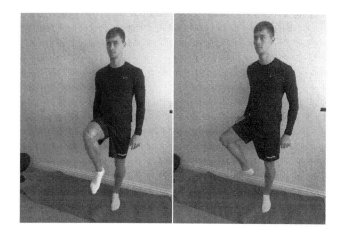

## HIIT 2 Exercises

**Lying Superman Hold** – Starting position: Picture 1 shows that you should lay down facing the floor with your arms slightly in front of you and your legs slightly apart while relaxed. Use your core and lower back to raise your arms and legs off the ground, hold this position for a split second before relaxing your muscles back into the starting position. Continue this for the time given, a great core exercise while working lower back and upper legs. Complete this as quick as you can to maintain the high heart rate.

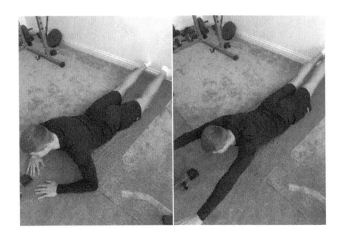

**Fast Feet** – Start standing with feet wider apart than usual and knees slightly bent. This is a fast-paced exercise so go through it slowly before picking up the pace. Keep your knees slightly bent and lift your left foot slightly off the ground (about an inch or so), then lower your left foot to the ground while simultaneously lifting your right foot off the ground. Keep alternating feet and do this at a fast pace. This exercise should wear you out and shoot your heart rate up – meaning you will burn fat. This may feel like sprinting on the spot.

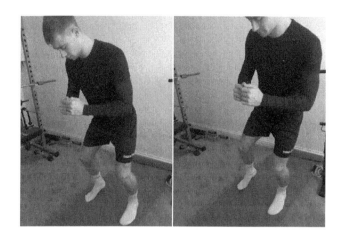

**Wall Sit** – This requires space in front of a wall. Start by standing with your back to the wall, squat down and sit with your back against the wall like the photos show below. Hold this position for the time given and you will certainly feel this in your glutes, calves and quads. After the previous exercises, the wall sit will hurt even more, it is all about mental toughness to get through it.

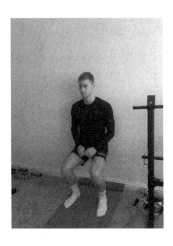

**Twist and Point** – Begin with hands and feet on the floor just like the press-up position. Then lift your left hand off the ground and twist your torso to face to the left so that your right hand is holding you up, while in that position raise your left hand as high as you can before bringing your hand back down to the ground to balance the weight of your body onto both arms. Then repeat this on your right side by holding your body up with your left hand and have your right arm is pointing up. Continue to switch between arms for the time period. This exercise will allow you to build endurance and strength in your triceps, shoulders and pectorals. Other muscles trained: upper back muscles and abdominals.

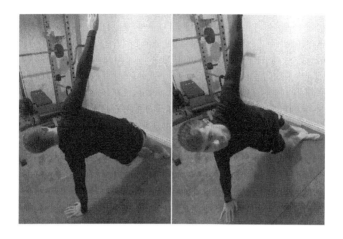

**Skipping** – This does not require a jump/skipping rope however if you have one you may as well use it. If you have the rope, then skip just like how you usually would – try to skip quickly and switch feet if you are skilled. If you do not have a rope then no worries, pretend that you are holding a rope and then skip – you may look slightly silly, but this exercise is still effective for burning calories and improves your foot-eye coordination. If you are pretending to skip, then do this at a face pace to keep your Heart Rate high.

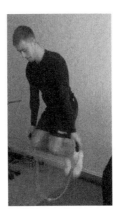

**Flutter Kicks** - Lay on the floor facing the sky with your hands behind your head - lifting your head and shoulder off the floor. Keep your legs straight and lift your left leg up while keeping your right leg slightly off the ground. From that position lower your left leg to the hovering position and raise your right leg up slightly like the second photo shows. Continue to move between the positions shown in the two photos below. This exercise is brilliant for strengthening back muscles, lower rectus abdominals and hip flexors. Don't let your feet touch the floor!

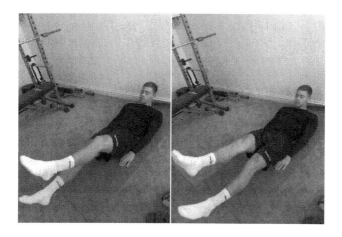

**Plank to Push up** – Start in the usual push-up position on your hands and tiptoes. From the push up position place your left forearm on the floor followed by your right forearm, do this while keeping your feet in the same position. Then as soon as your right forearm is placed on the floor you will be in the plank position. From this plank position get back into the push-up position by placing your left palm on the ground, then your right palm and finally push up with your arms. Continue to move from the two positions shown in the photos below. This exercise is great for building strength and endurance in your deltoids, pectorals, triceps and your rectus abdominals.

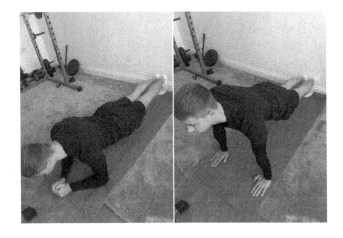

**Side Plank** – Start by laying down with your left forearm on the floor with the side of your left foot on the floor, look at the 1$^{st}$ photo for inspiration. Hold this position for the time given in the HIIT Circuit instructions before swapping to the right side. For the right-side plank, place your right forearm on the ground and the right side of your right foot on the ground while keeping your body off the floor (2nd photo). This exercise works your obliques and should make most of your body ache as it is the last exercise of the circuit.

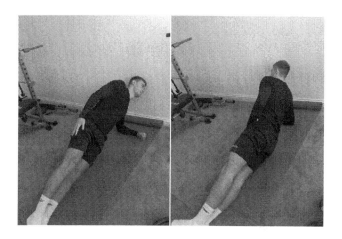

**HIIT 3 Exercises**

**Twist and point** – Previously Explained. Make sure you complete quicker reps to maintain the higher heart rate.

**Snake Push-ups** – These are brutal! Start in a high push-up position (photo 1), tiptoes on the floor with legs slightly bent, bum sticking up and your hands planted on the floor shoulder width apart. To complete a Snake Push-up: use your arms to lower your chest to the ground while simultaneously moving your chest slightly forwards to get to the position of photo 2. Then from that position push up through your arms to get to the final position where you should be ready to go again. This exercise is great for triceps, deltoids and pectorals, the angle at which you push up causes your muscles to exert more.

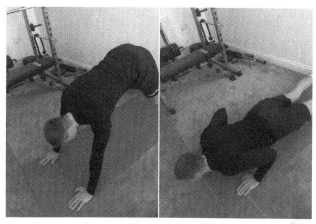

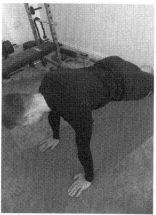

**Mountain Climbers** - Start with your hands and feet on the floor like you're in a push up position. Then while keeping your hands planted on the ground, bring your left knee to your chest. From this position (Photo 1), kick your left leg back to where it was in the push up position, while at the same time bringing your right knee to your chest. Continue to switch from the positions shown in both pictures below. Great exercise specific to burning belly fat.

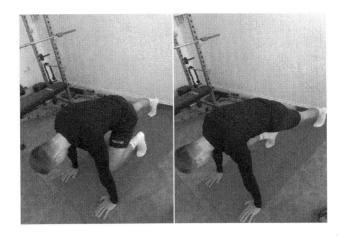

**Squat Jumps** – Firstly stand with your feet slightly wider than shoulder width apart and facing outwards. Then squat down by sitting back, shifting your weight into your heels while bending your knees, once you get as low down as you can, push up through your heels and toes to jump up explosively. Use your arms to help create momentum for your jump. Once you land the squat jump you should carry on squatting down and jumping up until your times up! Great for building strength mainly in quads, hamstrings, calves, glutes as well as lower back muscles and abdominals. Requires many different muscles to perform a jump meaning you will burn calories and improve explosive power. Try to get as many jumps as you can in the time provided.

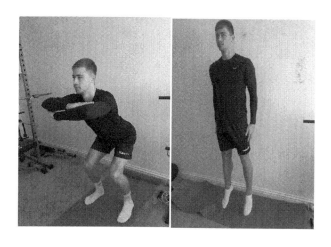

**Standing Side Crunch** – Begin by standing straight with your hands behind your head with fingers locked together. Use your hands to push your head down to the left while leaning to the left and raising your left knee (2nd photo), this should make you feel a slight burn in your obliques. Hold that position for a split second before lowering your left leg. Then lean to the right and raise your right knee to feel the same burn just this time on the other side (3rd photo). This exercise helps your improve balance and strengthen obliques. Complete quicker than usual to match the required heart rate.

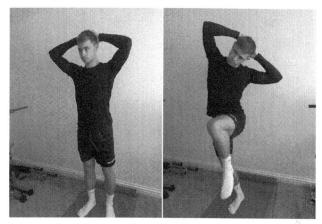

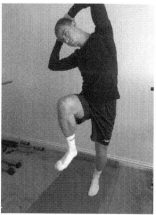

**Ali Shuffle** – Start with your left foot in front of your right and knees slightly bent (1$^{st}$ photo). Then hop off the ground slightly so you can bring your left foot back and your right foot forwards at the same time (2<sup>nd</sup> photo), when you land you should hop again straightaway and then shuffle your feet back to the starting position. Do this continuously so you are always swapping feet. A great cardiovascular activity that will improve foot-eye coordination and will give you fast feet. (If you have ankle weights knocking about then stick them on!) This exercise was made popular by the great Muhammad Ali and look how it helped him out. Get as many shuffles in as you can in the time given.

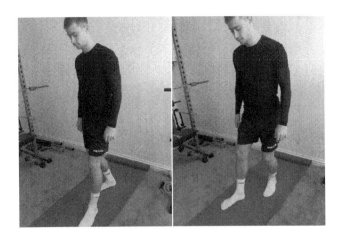

**Straight Punches** – Start by standing in a causal boxing stance, do this by placing your weak foot (pointing forwards) in front of your strong foot (which should face outwards) and hold your arms high with your fists clenched like the 1$^{st}$ photo shows below – always keep your knees slightly bent. To throw a left straight punch then simply extend your left arm out quickly until you cannot extend your arm anymore, which then you should instantly bring your arm back to the starting position – always keep a clenched fist and the punch should be like a snap. To throw a right straight punch, follow the same steps as the left straight punch but twist your body into the punch. My boxing book can always help you with form. The benefits from this include faster hands, will make you sweat and potentially hand eye coordination. Repeat left-right-left-right straight punches very quickly for the time period.

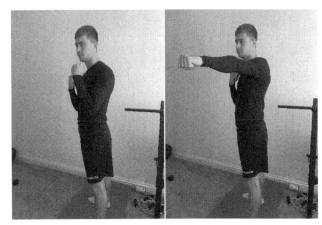

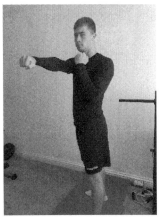

**Lunges with Twists**- From a standing position take one foot forward and keep the other foot planted, shift your weight onto the front leg and bend both legs. Once in the lunge position twist your body to the left (Picture 1) then to the right (Picture 2) using your arms and lower back then finally step back into a standing position. Works your legs and lower back. Also, remember to alternate the leg which you lunge froward with.

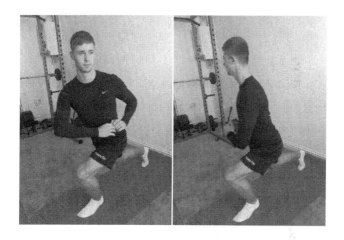

**Wall Sits** – Previously explained. Will be harder in this circuit due to the higher intensity causing your muscles to ache more, you sure will have strong legs if you stick to this.

**Twist Jumps** – Stand with feet slightly wider than shoulder width apart, drop into a squat while twisting your body and arms to the left. Then quickly swing your arms to the right to and use your lower back to twist your torso to the right while jumping up through your heels, so that you jump up and rotate 90 degrees clockwise in the air. Land the jump and repeat, change direction whenever you feel like it. Improves agility, flexibility in hips and leg strength. Complete quickly, get as many jumps in as possible.

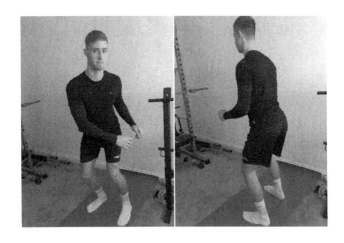

## VHIIT Exercises

**Half Squat Jumps** – Start in the position shown in the first photo, to do this place your feet shoulder-width apart and slightly bend your legs. From this position bend your knees a little bit to drop down into the half squat, then spring up through your heels to elevate slightly off the ground (Photo 2). Land from the jump in the position of photo 1, and you are good to repeat again and again. This exercise is great for getting a sweat on and also strengthens legs. These need to be performed very quickly, don't jump too high so you can get as many jumps as possible in the time.

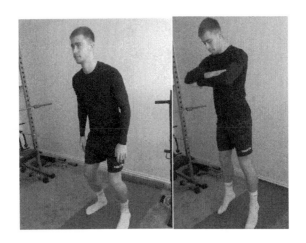

**Power Star** – This is like an explosive star jump. Start by standing with legs together, then bend your knees to bend down and touch your toes (1st photo), before quickly jumping straight up and raising your arms with side of you to appear as a star (Blurry 2nd Photo). On the way back down to the floor bring your arms back to your sides and legs together so you are ready to do another Power Star. Another great cardio exercise which mainly works the leg muscles, but is an entire body workout.

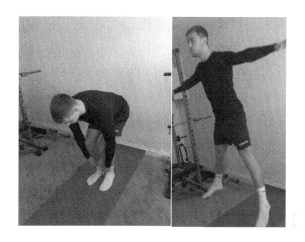

**Bicycle Crunches** – Previously Explained. Work faster.

**Mountain Climbers** – Previously Explained. Work Faster.

**Boxer Squat** – Begin by standing with feet facing slightly outwards and placed wider than shoulder width apart. Keep your hands up in a boxer guard (1st photo). Squat down by sitting back and bending your knees as far down as you can go. Then from the squat position push up through your heels back to the starting position and throw a straight left and a straight right punch (1-2). To punch, fully extend your arms your quickly in front of you one after the other then bring your arms back to the starting boxer guard position to go again. Remember to be quick!

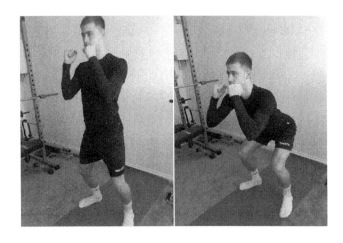

**Fast High Knees** – Start by standing in usual position but try to keep light on your feet. This needs to be fast paced: Firstly, lift your left knee as high as you can (1st photo), then lower your left foot to the ground while you raise your right knee as high as you can (2nd photo). Repeat this very quickly throughout the 30 seconds, it may feel like sprinting on the spot. Great cardio and will certainly burn many calories.

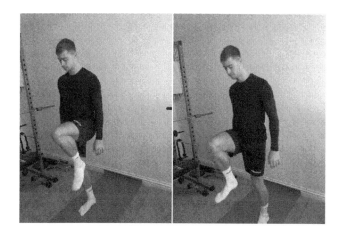

**100%**

**Fast Feet** - Previously explained, just now needs to be as fast as you possibly can.

**Burpee with Push-up** – Prepare yourself to do a burpee (previously explained), carry out the burpee but this time when you drop down into the push-up position instead of hopping your feet closer to your hands to get back up, you should complete a push-up by lowering your chest to the ground and pushing back up with your arms (Transition from photo 2 to photo 3). After you complete the push-up then you can bring your feet to your hands to jump up. Try to be quick with the push up to maintain high Heart Rate.

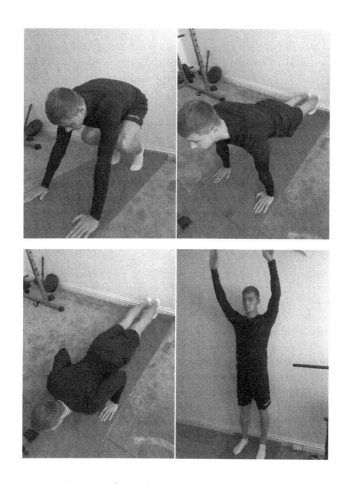

**Diamond Push-up** – A very tough push-up indeed. Start with hands and feet on the floor like how you would usually start for many floor exercises, however, bring your hands closer together and into a diamond shape like the first photo shows below. Always keep your hands and feet planted to the ground while you use your arms to lower your chest to your hands, from that position (photo 2) push back up with your arms. This kind of push-up is great for strengthening triceps, also strengthens pectorals and deltoids.

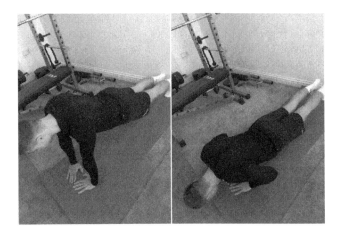

**Side Plank** – Previously explained, will be harder due to higher intensity of other exercises.

**Reverse Crunches** – Lay flat on your back facing the ceiling/sky to get into the starting position. Always keep your hands planted on the floor either side of you for support. Then bring your knees as far as possible towards your face while keeping your feet together (Photo 1). When your knees are near your chest, extend your legs forwards while keeping them off the floor (Photo 2). Continue to switch between these two positions below using your core and lower back to move your legs. This exercise works the full length of the rectus abdominal muscle, making this the most efficient exercise for getting a six-pack.

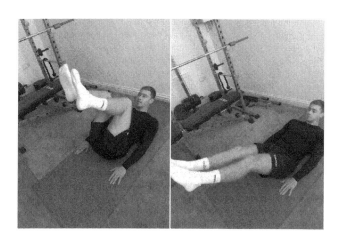

**Squat Thrusts** – Start with hands and feet on the floor like in a high push up position (1st Photo). Remember to always keep your hands planted in the same position and hop both your feet together forwards and back repeatedly (Photo 2 to Photo 1), when hopping forwards aim to bring your knees close to your chest and when you hop back just get into the starting position. Try to take most of your bodyweight with your arms. This exercise is brilliant for burning belly fat.

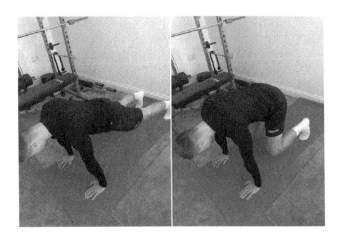

**Snake Push-ups** – Previously explained. You will have to give it everything for this exercise, I imagine that you will be absolutely shattered but you have to keep going.

## Warmup Exercise Descriptions

**Jog on Spot** – Not much to say, just like you are running but not in any direction.

**Knee Hugs** – From a standing position, raise your left knee to your chest and hold it for a few seconds before letting go and swapping to perform the hug with your right leg.

**Sexy Circles** – Stand tall with your feet wide apart and keep your hands on your hips. For the 30 seconds, proceed to rotate your hips in circles using your legs and lower back to do so. This exercise loosens up your hips and groin, remember to spend

15 seconds going clockwise, 15 seconds anti-clockwise and make sure you look good doing it!

**Arm Extension Hold** – In a standing or sitting position, raise both arms up as high as you can (so that your palms are facing up) and lock your fingers together. From that position roll your shoulders up to extend your arms further and push up through your fingers, hold this for 10-15 seconds to give your arms a good stretch then you should stretch again after a slight rest. Overall, stretch twice in the 30 second period.

**Ankle Rolls** – Stand with feet shoulder width apart. Raise your left heel so that your tiptoes are on the floor and have your right foot planted on the floor, then rotate your left ankle clockwise using your tiptoes. After 15 or so seconds, switch foot so your right foot is on its tiptoes then rotate that for 15 seconds. This stretches the ligaments, muscles and tendons in and around your ankle.

**Lateral Split Squat Stretch** – Start by standing in a wide stance with your feet flat and your toes pointing straight ahead. Squat down towards the left while bending your left leg and keeping your right leg straight, hold this for 10-15 seconds before standing up and bending to the right to stretch your alternative leg. This stretches most of the major leg muscles and should be done slowly.

**High Kick Outs** – This requires plenty of space to complete. From a standing position you will need to kick out in front of you with your left leg while your right foot is planted, try to get your left leg as high as you can while keeping it extended. Once your foot gets as high as possible, bring your left leg down and repeat the kick out with your right leg. Continue to kick and swap legs for the 30 seconds. This yet again stretches leg muscles and uses your core.

**Heel Flicks** – From a standing position, kick your left foot back towards your bum while keeping your right foot on it tiptoes. Then as you bring your left foot down towards the floor you should kick back your right foot towards your bum. Continue to flick your feet towards your bum in the order of left foot, then right foot for a minute. This will loosen up your leg muscles and get your heart beating quicker.

**Child Pose** – Start by kneeling on the floor. From that position place both hands on the floor in front of you and continue to stretch your arms out as far as they can go. Eventually you will get to a point where you can't extend your arms any further, hold that position for 10 seconds before relaxing and going back to the kneeling position. Repeat that twice in the 30 second period to stretch your lower back.

**Calves Stretch** – Find a wall with a bit of open space in front of it. Stand in front of the wall and place your left foot on the wall, press down on the wall with your left tiptoes to stretch your calf, you should feel this burning sensation if you are doing it correctly. Hold that for 10 to 15 seconds before stretching your right calf.

**Hamstring Stretch** - To stretch your left leg: Start by standing up straight, then bend your right knee slightly while extending your left leg so your left heel is on the floor and your toes are pointing upwards. Hold this stretch for 10-15 seconds. Then switch leg by repeating the steps but alternatively. If you don't feel anything the press down with your hands onto your bent knee as this force will certainly stretch the hamstrings.

**Chest Stretch** – This can be done standing or sitting. Puff your chest out by inhaling heavily, then keep your arms behind your back. Your arms behind your back should be crossed and you need to try to touch your right elbow with your left hand and your left elbow with your right hand, as you are reaching your arms across, you will be stretching your chest. Hold the stretch for 10 seconds before having a break and going again.

**Side Lunge** – Begin by standing with feet shoulder width apart. Twist your left foot 90 degrees anticlockwise then lunge forwards in that direction while keeping your right foot planted. Hold that lunge for 10 to 15 seconds before stepping back in and rotating your left foot back to the starting position. Remember to do both sides by rotating your right foot 90 degrees clockwise then lunging forwards in that direction.

**Backpedalling** – As I understand many of you will be working out in a limited space, here is an alternative method on how to complete. From a standing position jog forwards a couple of steps, after that you will want to bend your knees and get low to run backwards around 4 steps (face the same direction just run backwards). Without sounding too crazy, you will continue to run back and forth for the time given.

**5 Burpees** – Previously explained. Just do 5 burpees in your own time as the final heart raiser before getting into the workout. Should take from 30 to 60 seconds, don't complete these burpees too quickly as it's a warmup.

## Cooldown Exercise Descriptions

**Light Jog on Spot** - Just a slow gentle jog to lower your heart rate, which I imagine is pounding out of your chest after a HIIT Circuit.

**Lunges** – This is like the exercise "Lunges and Twist", without the twist. So, for this cooldown activity, lunge forwards with your left leg from a standing position and hold that lunge for 10 to 15 seconds before stepping back. Then lunge forwards with your right foot and hold for the remaining time. This will stretch the major leg muscles and lower back.

**Close the Gates** – Open and Close the Gates previously explained in this chapter. You will just need to complete the second part of that exercise, for example you will start with your left knee raised 90 degrees to the left to which you will use your hip to rotate your knee clockwise until it is directly in front of you. Make sure to close the gates slowly to increase the range of motion on your hips. Also remember to close the gate for both legs.

**Seated Spinal Twists** – Begin by sitting down with your back straight. For the 30 seconds you will need to slowly rotate your body from left to right using your lower back and arms.

**Neck Rolls** – A very nice dynamic stretch. Can be done standing or sitting. Roll your head clockwise around your shoulders using your neck very slowly for 15 seconds, then roll your head anticlockwise for the remaining time.

**Calf Raises** – Start in the usual standing position but be on your tiptoes. Simply press up through your tiptoes slowly as high as you can go, once you reach that position slowly lower your heels to the floor. Continue to repeat that motion slowly to feel the burning sensation in your lower legs.

**Bicep Stretch** – To do this simply stretch out your left arm with the palm facing up. With your right hand, you should push down on the palm of the stretched-out arm. You should feel your forearm and bicep being stretched. Repeat on the other arm.

**Shake off Arms and Legs** – It is what it says. Spend a few seconds shaking your left leg off with your foot off the ground to increase blood flow, the do the same with your right leg. Keep both your arms down and shake them off gently for the time being as well. Not much else to say apart from give them a good shake.

## Benefits of Training Muscles

Throughout this chapter, I have included the muscles that are worked during each exercise (for most of them at least). For most people that may not mean anything, so here is a section to explain why training each particular muscle is important and can help you in many ways.

**Calf** – This is the muscle that is found at the back of the leg below the knee, made up of two smaller muscles: Soleus and Gastrocnemius. This is a major leg muscle which supports your upper legs and body. Exercises that require for the calf to be used will make the calf stronger over time. Having strong calves is great because it allows for you to run faster, run for longer, jump higher, keep a more consistent running pace and can easily support your body if the rest of your muscles become heavier.

**Quadriceps** – These are located at the front of the leg above the knee. You engage your quads for most of the day, whether that's by walking or standing or biking then you will be using your quads, so they are important as they keep you moving. Having strong and flexible quads will boost your knee function because it will take most the stress away from the knees, your knees without any other muscular support are more likely to be damaged under stress from body weight (having weak quads is likely to end up knee osteoporosis). Having strong and flexible quads will also make daily activities like walking, running and standing easier for your entire body.

**Hamstrings** – These are tendons that are at the back of the thigh that attach the thigh muscle to the bone. This muscle is usually engaged during activities that involve bending the knee, for example: running, jumping or climbing. Stronger Hamstrings will allow you to achieve better speed, power and agility with exercise and many sports. Plus, having weak hamstrings will damage your knees. It is important to stretch your hamstrings out at the end of a workout because that will prevent them shortening and losing elasticity. Having strong hamstrings will also reduce strain on other ligaments or tendons, which reduces injury.

**Glutes** – The glutes are found in the buttocks and are considered one of the strongest muscles in the body. The benefits of having strong glutes include increased athletic performance as you can run faster, jump higher and become more agile. Also helps with injury prevention because strong glutes will reduce the strain on the lower back muscles, knees and leg muscles. Overall, having strong glutes will keep your body functioning to the best of its ability.

**Biceps** – Biceps are found in the front of your upper arm. The advantages of having strong biceps include improved bone density, a higher resistance to injury, greater upper body strength, bigger arms and will help you achieve more power in sports that involve throwing, tossing or swinging. Although biceps are difficult to engage without equipment, it still can be done.

**Triceps** – Found along the back of the upper arms. They allow for movement in your shoulders and elbows. Triceps are engaged when we straighten or lock our elbows – an example of this is by pushing objects away from us or exercises like push ups. Having strong triceps will help build upper body strength, which is helpful for stabilizing your shoulders, will increase your pushing power, will allow you to build larger arms which may make you appear more attractive. String Triceps will also help you with many sports and activities like tennis.

**Pectoral** – Located in the chest and is made up of four muscles. These muscles are commonly known as 'pecs', the pecs connect the front of the of the chest with the bones of the upper arms and shoulders. The pectoral muscles are used to move the arms and also moves the ribcage during deep breathing. Having strong pectoral muscles brings many benefits like:

- Can improve posture.
- Increases the strength in your back muscles – the back muscles are later explained.
- Increases upper body strength.
- Improving your ability to push things.
- Can improve your ability to perform swinging movements.
- Finally, it can allow for an improved appearance of the chest.

**Shoulders** – The deltoid muscles are the muscles that form the rounded contour of the shoulder. Having strong shoulders will make arm movements easier like throwing, tossing, pulling or pushing. It also helps with injury prevention, if you have weak shoulders but like to train pecs and triceps, then your shoulders are likely to get injured because the deltoids won't be able to cope with the workload that the other two muscles can handle. Of course, there is an appearance factor, it is likely that you will appear more attractive with bigger and wider shoulders.

**Upper Back** – Many muscles are involved in the upper back. There is not much point of me listing all the muscles, but you may have heard of lats, traps and rhomboids. Each muscle in your upper back has a job to keep the body held upright and allow for trunk movements. Below you can find a list of benefits that come with a strong upper back:

- Prevents injury as the back muscles take the stress away from the shoulders.
- Improves upper body strength – will allow you to pull heavier objects towards you.
- Increased support for neck and shoulders which will reduce potential neck and back pain.
- Helps maintain a good posture.
- Back muscles are the second strongest muscle group in the body, training those muscles expands plenty of energy which helps your body maintain high energy levels.
- Strong backs look good. (A common feature with all muscles)

**Lower Back** – Many muscles make up the lower back. Just like the upper back there is no point listing all the individual muscles but they allow us to stand and lift objects up. The benefits of a strong back are almost identical to the benefits that come with a strong upper back. The only differences being that strong lower back muscles can strengthen the core, leg and arm muscles.

I want this book to give you as much information as possible and I hope the information provided on the benefits that come with strengthening each muscle will encourage you to include more HIIT Circuits in your training routine. The most common benefit of building up all these muscles is that you will become a stronger, faster, and bigger individual. If you are starting off overweight, then don't think that building lean muscle will make you go up a size because you will just be building your perfect physique for when you do burn all the fat surrounding it. Building lean muscle mass has a huge correlation with injury prevention.

Plus, for you ladies that think building muscle will make you unattractive, don't stress about it because these exercises are hardly going to make you look masculine overnight and it's not a bad thing to be strong. Lean muscle mass will keep you looking toned and brings you all the benefits, so it's not something to miss out on.

# Chapter 8 – Improvise, Adapt and Overcome

As I am sure you are all aware, 2020 has been unpredictable to say the least. With all the unfortunate events that have occurred, many people had to change the way they live – the most common difference being that many people have spent much longer inside. While most people just accept the change that they're not happy with or bored of, some people decide to improvise, adapt and overcome the change.

By that phrase I mean that people use their creativity to try carry on their normal life from home so that they are not wasting any valuable time, because you do only have one life at the end of the day which makes our time precious. This chapter is focused on mindset more than anything, providing lots of motivation to help you find your inner determination to get things done! Yes, I agree that relaxing at home for a couple days is nice, but for a month? Is that not boring? Just watching the same crap over and over again while making no progress towards any of your goals, because I'd say that is a terrible use of time.

I want this chapter not to only help you mentally to reach your fitness goals, but just you help you out generally. Mental health is a big concern worldwide and the problems caused by lockdown and isolation are putting people in a bad place. Being stuck inside with a lack of entertainment, facing loneliness or having no access to gyms really isn't great for your mental wellbeing. I want you to be able to look back at this lockdown period, or even if you are reading this in 2030, I want you to look back at a hard time in your life and feel proud of how you dealt with it.

**Improvise**

Instead of accepting that you can't do something because you find it too hard or there are restrictions holding you back, you have to break down the problem bit by bit to discover what is that is specifically causing you the problem. For example, with getting into a training routine it may be that you cannot wake up early in the morning to complete your workout – it is now your job to think about why you cannot wake up early. Is it because you went to be too late the night before? Is it because you can't find the motivation to get out of bed in the morning? Or it may be a little thing, did you forget to set an alarm?

Once you ask yourself these questions you may then realise why you can't do it. This improvising step is about finding where the problem lies and will hopefully show you what you can do to solve the problem in a way that is specific to you. Your problem won't be solved if somebody just says, "Well just wake up and get out of bed earlier". It is better if somebody asks you those questions and uses your answers to suggest solutions such as: "Remember to set an alarm for when you want to wake up", "Try to get to sleep earlier the night before", "C'mon, you need to get up because if you don't then you will not reach your goal". Of course, it is easier said than done, doing something about it has a much bigger impact towards reaching greatness.

The problem and solution there is quite concise, and I know that there are many other reasons why it is a struggle to get into a training routine. But that doesn't mean this method won't work for your problems or difficulties.

Now, it is most likely that you are going to be the only person asking yourself these questions and answering yourself, which may seem a bit crazy, but stay with me. It is much easier to feel motivated by having a PT or person there persuading you to get stuff done, but as it is likely you will be on this journey alone so that is why you must learn to motivate yourself. You will be the only person to ask yourself the questions on why you failed and come up with solutions on how to win.

Plus, there are many solutions for each problem, it's all about thinking outside the box. If you really don't like the idea of waking up early to complete a HIIT circuit, then you don't have to. Instead, you can complete the HIIT Circuit later on in the day, as long as you have a plan that works for you so that you don't have to make any sacrifices like waking up early. Please note this may result in other issues, but I am hoping you'll learn how to overcome them with this guide.

## Adapt

This is the next stage of the mental mindset to go with fitness or anything really. I would like to say that this stage is where you go for it, this is where you make your first mark towards greatness. This may be the hardest step out of the three.

Sticking with the previous example which was all about not being able to wake up early enough to exercise, to adapt to solving the problem you would have to start making changes to what you do. For example, you would want to set alarm, go to bed earlier the night before and force yourself out of bed. That's the hardest part because once you are out of bed your body will get out of that resting state, all it leaves you to do now is complete the exercise and get on with the rest of your day. I use this example because it was something I previously struggled with, I found that in order to wake up earlier I had to leave my phone halfway across my room, so I had to physically get out of bed to click snooze – once I was up, there was no point me going back to sleep and that's how I got through my day.

You may find that the first time you do that something different to overcome your problem that the rest of your day may be much more difficult than imagined– for example if you exercise early in the morning for the first time you may find yourself struggling more to complete the exercise. This is because you are not used to the change as of yet and the overcome stage is what will help you bypass the struggle, the only way to get around this to keep going again and again. You may start to see that overtime it gets easier and it will be worth it in the long run. You can apply the adapt method to anything. You need to give your body time to adjust, it doesn't all happen overnight!

## Overcome

The final step, the one that is achieved by consistency. The definition of overcome is when you succeed in dealing with (a problem or difficulty). You will reach the stage of overcoming once you are in a position when the thing that was stopping you reach your goal (for example not being able to wake up in the morning to exercise), is no longer a problem, just instead something that you complete comfortably (now being able to wake up on time every day and being prepared for the workout).

You can overcome any personal problem, but it is important that you stick to a routine to do so. The longer that you put off dealing with a challenge the harder it gets each day to build up courage/motivation to tackle that same challenge – in other words the longer you spend hesitating the more likely you are to give up. Giving up isn't an option, it doesn't let you achieve anything apart from regret.

In order to overcome your problem(s), you must follow the previous two steps "Improvise" – to discover what is causing your problem and how to get around it, "Adapt" – to start trying the method to get around the problem and now finally you must "Overcome" – to consistently get around the problem until eventually it is no longer a problem. To explain this, I will stick with the example of not waking up on time to train. To overcome this situation then you will want to do all you can to make sure that you wake up on time. This can be done by setting an alarm for when you want to wake up, by going to sleep earlier the night before and pushing yourself mentally to get up. If you get into a habit of following them 3 solutions, then eventually it will all become natural, after a while it won't even cross your mind that you are waking up earlier to exercise because your body clock will adapt to the new training time and you will feel great about yourself.

So, the best way to put it is that if you want to succeed then you will need to find something that works and stick to it. I am unaware of what is stopping you exercise or any of your other problems, that's why I hope for this to help you find your own solutions to your problems. I believe you can use this advice for any challenges you face, it seriously helps and is quite simple. You see many motivational tips for fitness which involve all these complications, but this simple technique will prevent you wasting time and feeling down.

If this doesn't help you overcome your problems to do with fitness, then you should probably look for personal trainers as support – there is only so much that I can write in this book and by email. I physically cannot be there to support you, that is why I want to point you in the direction of where to reach support because I want the best for you. There are many Fitness groups on Facebook you can join, or you can even contact your local gym to get into contact with a PT.

## Short term Discomfort, Long term Gain

Living comfortably is a real privilege that many people get to experience every day, let's be honest most of us (including myself) take living comfortably for granted. It is only when we go through a period of stress or discomfort that we wish that we could go back to how we were living beforehand. But many people across the world don't live comfortably, which is a huge problem, but sadly it is just how it is and will take years to sort out. Although, there is limit to how I can help people in discomfort (donation is my best option), this makes me think about how people that live in struggle are generally more driven and are mentally prepared for anything that comes their way. You often hear these 'Rags to Riches' stories about people who had absolutely nothing and worked their ass off to get to the top – Manny Pacquiao is a great example.

I am not saying that you should ditch your comfortable life just to increase your chances of becoming successful. But instead, you should consider putting your body/mind in a short period of discomfort. Why? This is because discomfort to the mind or body is something that we are not used to, this makes your body or mind slowly adapt to the change which then allows for growth. You ever heard of the term, no pain no gain? This saying is exactly what discomfort will bring you, that short period of physical or mental pain will make you physically and mentally stronger in the future.

There are endless ways on how you can get into a position of discomfort, whether that is staying for an extra hour of work, running an extra mile, or waking up earlier each week. Each method of discomfort will make you grow towards your goals and of course I will use fitness to prove this. So, if you really want to reach your goals, you have to sacrifice your comfort for it. I think that is a fair deal because a period of discomfort every now and then will help you develop a strong mindset to hit any target you set yourself.

You must think long term. I understand it is hard to turn down short term comfort, like a glass of wine or a chocolate bar, because it is nice. Remember that a chocolate bar will do absolutely no good for you and you know that, but if you stick to your healthy diet then in the long run you will achieve your fitness goal and you don't have to completely cut out nice unhealthy food – just limit it to once a week and stick to the limits.

Living comfortably is likely to make you lazy, unmotivated and you will not make progress to life towards your goals. Unless your goal is to be a couch potato! So, look for periods of short-term discomfort, it will do you some good.

Short term discomfort links to progressive overload in a way that you are pushing your body harder during exercise to make that fitness gain over time. But this chapter doesn't always have to help you with fitness, whether you find talking to new people uncomfortable, whether you are scared to put your name out there or whatever the reason is, you should just get it done. It may be embarrassing or wrong at first, causing discomfort, however you will learn from mistakes and come back better and more confident. I believe confidence to be the best driving factor to help to reach your goals, and you can build your confidence through short term discomfort!

## Exercise is Good for Your Brain

The physical benefits of exercise are easier to spot and have already been discussed. Although the physical benefits are nice, I believe the mental benefits to massively outweigh the physical benefits. I love to exercise because I feel great afterwards, I would never have known why I feel so good after a workout without research. Below is a list of mental benefits exercise can bring:

- Physical Activity increases the endorphin levels – endorphins are the 'Happy' chemicals in the brain which make you feel great. This mood booster can decrease the symptoms of depression and anxiety.

- Decreased Stress – Increasing your heart rate over a short period can reverse stress induced brain damage by stimulating the production of neurohormones. Your body will be able to respond to stress better, which contributes towards feeling happy.

- Brain Boost – Exercise can boost your brain power in several ways to improve memory and build intelligence. Studies show that physical activity on mice and humans will create new brain cells and improve overall brain performance. So, if you have exams to study for, get your HIIT circuits in!

- Increased Confidence – Although the last few paragraphs are here to help you build up your confidence, you will find yourself much more confident once you start making progress towards your goals and start looking good. Be proud of what you have achieved and show off, it's the little things like being able to do 10 burpees without huffing and puffing - while 6 months previously you couldn't even do 5 burpees. This confidence will come naturally, enjoy it!

I think that is enough to persuade you to exercise even if you haven't got a proper goal to work towards. Think of this as a bonus for you reaching your goal, or as your actual goal. With that said, let's move on to more motivation because you can never get enough.

## More Motivation

I want for this chapter to a point in which can be read over and over again due to the valuable information included, for this chapter in particular I want for you to re-read this when you haven't got the drive, or you can't be bothered to lay out your fitness mat and complete a HIIT Circuit. This sub-chapter contains a few motivational tips that are different to the ones included in the previous books and will help you get up and get on with it.

**Have a Setback Plan** – This is where you plan out how to deal with a possible setback like an injury or illness. As unfortunate as a setback is, it should still be planned for because there is always a possibility that you may get injured and you need to know how to deal with the setback. From each injury you pick up you will learn something, once you feel pain you will naturally think back to the potential reasons for the injury - whether it's because you forgot to warm up and you overstretched a muscle during an exercise causing a strain or you were wearing incorrect footwear and slipped on the floor causing a damaged elbow. Once you are injured, you will make a mental note to not do that again, as you know it will cause pain.

A setback plan can contain plenty of information for when you do get injured. Firstly, when you get injured you should be able to focus on what you can and can't do, if it is a serious injury and your doctor tells you to take time off exercise then please listen to them, but if it is a less minor injury then think of ways you can get exercise in without using the injured body part and stick to your previous routine as it can be hard to get back into routine after being out of one for so long – even just walking every day is still exercise. Secondly, focus on your mental health. This is the number one priority because injury can cause stress which isn't needed. Ways in which you can keep a positive mental include surrounding yourself with positive people, doing the things you like (unless it will make your setback worse), getting outside the house and I am sure that you know what helps you best in that situation. Thirdly – don't rush back into training, take your time to let your illness/injury fully go away/heal before training again because if you exercise while unwell or injured it is likely to make matters worse. Finally, you should be able to find rehab exercises which should be gentle and allow for the injured part of your body to be strengthened slowly but surely, so that the rate in which your body can recover from injury increases, meaning that you'll be exercising before you know it.

In the actual setback plan, you should keep a brief note somewhere of what has been suggested previously in a way that is specific to you, so that if you do become injured then you will avoid the negatives that come with the injury - the negatives which may end with further set back and poor mental state – and get back into training as soon as possible. While you are following your setback plan, you should also stick to your healthy diet plan as your body needs the energy to repair, don't let your good habits slip.

**Competition** – Having a competition amongst friends which is based on reaching fitness goals or any goals is very motivational. As a competitive person myself, I like winning competitions between friends and family even if they are pointless. So, a competition between friends to see who can get their body fat percentage to 5% first, or whatever your goals are, will be very helpful because it will make exercising seem like it has more of a purpose for you and it makes it more fun. This gives you a chance to beat your friends and claim bragging rights!

**Routine** – A routine is a sequence of actions followed in a sequence. Getting into a training routine is highly motivating because it is something that your body can naturally adjust to. Exercising at certain times in the day, eating 5 times a day with meals 3 hours apart and getting sufficient sleep. Once your body naturally adjusts to your new diet and training plan then it will get easier and feel natural. They say that 3 weeks builds a habit so once you get past the first 3 weeks, you will start completing HIIT Circuits 5 or 6 times a week without thinking about it. If you have to miss a day of training because of unexpected events, then don't stress about it just make sure you don't break your routine for any longer because it is much easier to maintain a routine than break it and have to get back into one.

**Learn Positive Self-talk** – Think about when a coach or trainer tells you not to give up and keep training, it helps you keep going right? If I was coaching you 1 to 1 then I would be more than happy to support you in this way, but I don't think me writing "C'mon, you can do it!" is as effective as me being there physically to support you. That's why you should learn to encourage yourself, there are many ways in which you can do this – personally I tell myself during a workout "I already know what giving up feels like, so I want to know what it feels like if I don't". Now it doesn't mean you have to say that out loud, that may be a bit awkward in a gym, but think of a way that prevents you giving up, just like how a coach would.

Other motivational tips are in this book and the last two books of this series, some may be more hidden than others, but the idea is that you have much more motivation than you need! Please don't use this motivation to push yourself way too hard, I want you to still stick to your routine as overtraining is linked with a higher chance of injury.

## The Comfort Zone

To put this in the best way, you need to push your body to its maximum limit in order to grow towards your goal and see the results. HIIT isn't meant to be easy after all. Although there is something that you should be careful with, and that is pushing yourself way too far out of the comfort zone to the danger zone. As you know, you are likely to be injured if you overtrain but at the same time you need to overtrain to make the gains. That may be very confusing because it's a recipe for injury, but at your fitness level, your body will be able to cope with training at exhaustion for a short period of time – this period of time is where you make the gains. It is only if you try to exercise at exhaustion for a long period of time that you will be at a high risk of injury.

This is something to be careful about, because like mentioned before there is a limit to how far you can get out of your comfort zone. For an example in term of a HIIT Circuit: you could train the HIIT Circuit for an extra 20 seconds, in which you will leaving your comfort zone as you will be at the exhaustion level and this will allow for muscles to be slightly damaged, so that they repair and grow back stronger (causing growth). However, you should not try to train the HIIT Circuit for an extra 2 minutes because your body will be at the point of exhaustion for too long which is very likely to end with a muscle being strained (causing setback). To sum it up nicely, short term discomfort = growth, long term discomfort = danger zone = injury.

I hope that I have helped with this, I am very big on fitness inspiration and I hope to create more in the future to help more people. You may want to read this chapter a couple of times to cement this knowledge in your brain, if you don't agree with any of these tips please let me know in the reviews as I am always looking for ways to improve the quality of my books!

# Chapter 9 – Keeping Fit for Life

I have done all I can to help you, it's now your turn to take action with the information that this book provides. Usually at this point, I would say that there is another book that continues from where this is left off, however there is not a next book to this series. There is only so much I can offer, and I don't want to keep repeating myself across these books.

I guess if you have a good prior experience with exercise then you will have a general idea of how you are going to reach your fitness goal. If you are unsure how you are going to reach your goal, then use the six-week training plan from the previous books and use that to get into a routine until you can follow a training plan that satisfies your training requirements. If you are wanting to increase lean muscle mass, don't train circuits that include cardiovascular exercises only as that will only contribute to you losing weight, instead have a mixture of muscular exercises and cardiovascular exercises like squats, push-ups, high knees and so on.

If you are in a position where you cannot complete a HIIT Circuit, then your goal is to complete a HIIT Circuit. Once you reach your goals, that is not a good place to stop, set another one like lowering body fat percentage so you always have something to work towards. The idea is that you should know what you want to achieve, and you should know what will get you there, the hardest part is actually doing it. The previous chapter on motivation should be made easily accessible for you so that if you ever reach a point of struggle you can re-read that chapter for that motivation boost.

As you have made it to the end, I just want to share a secret. This book series was not just a Circuit Training series, the original series was Published last August and contained 4 books. These books were honestly poor, they were around 6,000 words long and each book was completely different, although still under the category of Circuit Training. The books were based on Circuit Training for Beginners (I changed that book and re-published it), Circuit Training - Muscular Strength (Unsavable), Circuit Training – Endurance Training (This one was a load of waffle) and finally Further Circuit Training – HIIT Circuits, which is now this book that has been renamed High Intensity Circuit Training. I managed to turn two books out of that series into this much better series (if I say so myself), the reviews allowed me to make these improvements and that these mistakes are just a part of learning.

So, if you keep making mistakes just like my atrocious book series then just break it down, realise what you are doing wrong and work on improving it – just like I have done with these books. This book series is not perfect by all means, but it is much better and can provide value to readers. Use this as motivation for when things go wrong.

# Conclusion

You have made it to the end of "High Intensity Circuit Training" and I hope this book has either motivated you, has had a positive impact towards your training routine, had a positive effect on your diet, made you learn something new or brought you joy.

This book being the last of the Circuit Training for Weight Loss, I hope that you have all the knowledge to burn fat whether it is to lose weight, lower body fat percentage or exercise for the mental benefits. Below is a brief summary of this book for a brief recap and so it can help you break down the book, so you know which parts to refer to when you need a recap of the information.

This book starts with chapter 1, an introductory chapter to explain what HIIT Circuits are and how they work, which shows the foundations of using circuit training in your fitness routine. Chapter 2 is focused on diet and nutrition and this goes through all the essential nutrients, the structure of a high protein diet, why a high protein diet is most efficient for fat burning, information on the metabolism and the importance of energy. Chapter 3 is all about things that can be done to enhance your training, including training tips, goal setting, injury prevention and progressive overload.

Chapter 4 is more aimed at those who may be experienced with exercise but still want to give HIIT a real good go because HIIT is considered the most effective fat burning training method, this chapter helps those who are not up to the level of HIIT work their way up to completing a HIIT Circuit. Chapter 5 contains the warmups and a cooldown that is used before and after each circuit. Chapter 6 contains the good stuff - the HIIT circuits, there are 5 HIIT Circuits all at different difficulties to provide you with variety.

Chapter 7, this contains the exercise descriptions and a photo for every exercise included in all the circuits. Not only this but there is also a section which explains the benefits of training each muscle to help you understand how the body works and why exercise is important. Chapter 8 is all about motivation where I go into detail about short term discomfort, talk about developing a determined mindset and other positives that exercise can bring to your mental state. Chapter 9, the final chapter which is just a point to suggest how you can use the information in this book to take your training to the next level do you can hit your goals on time.

That's it from me, it's now up to you. Don't forget to check out the Circuit Training Weight Loss Bundle, many benefits in there you can't miss out on!

# My Books

## The Chump to Champ Collection

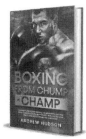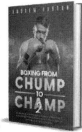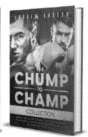

## Circuit Training for Weight Loss

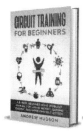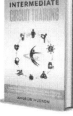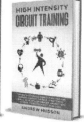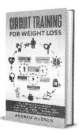

# Reference Page

*Dec Beales - Model for the Exercise Demonstrations.*

https://www.instagram.com/dec.beales/

*Your Free Gift – The Circuit Training Weight Loss Bundle.*

*https://hudsonandrew.activehosted.com/f/33*

*Join the Facebook Community.*

https://www.facebook.com/groups/workoutforweightloss

*Follow my Facebook Page.*

https://www.facebook.com/andrewhudsonbooks1

*Email me for extra support.*

andrew@hudsonandrew.com

A.A. (2018a). *Getting a fast metabolism*. Healthline. https://www.healthline.com/nutrition/get-a-fast-metabolism#what-it-is

A.B. (2019a). *Training tips*. Bodybuilding. https://www.bodybuilding.com/fun/10-best-training-tips-ever.htm

A.P. (2017a). *Caffeine before exercise*. Time. https://time.com/4842065/coffee-before-workout-caffeine/#:~:text=Caffeine%20can%20shift%20muscles%20to,its%20efficiency%20in%20generating%20power

*Benefits of strong hamstrings*. (2017). Atlaswearables. https://atlaswearables.com/blogs/atlas/the-benefits-of-strong-stretchy-hamstrings#:~:text=Strong%20hamstrings%20will%20help%20you,various%20ligaments%2C%20including%20the%20ACL

*Coping with injury*. (2016). Bodyshotperformance. https://www.bodyshotperformance.com/how-to-cope-with-injuries-and-setbacks-in-your-training/

D.B. (2018b). *Benefits of stretching*. Healthline. https://www.healthline.com/health/benefits-of-stretching

D.B. (2018c). *How to measure body fat*. Healthline. https://www.healthline.com/health/how-to-measure-body-fat#:~:text=To%20calculate%20body%20fat%20percentage%2C%20add%20your%20waist%20and%20hip,circumference%20value%20would%20be%2053

*Discomfort promotes growth*. (2018). Skilledatlife. http://www.skilledatlife.com/why-discomfort-is-good-and-a-sign-of-growth/#:~:text=It%20is%20a%20valuable%20opportunity,she%20can%20achieve%20almost%20anything.&text=The%20discomfort%20we%20feel%20while,are%20getting%20stronger%20and%20healthier

E.K.L. (2017b). *Glucose*. Healthline.

https://www.healthline.com/health/glucose

*Foods for better brainpower*. (n.d.). Health.Harvard.

Retrieved 2018, from

https://www.health.harvard.edu/mind-and-

mood/foods-linked-to-better-brainpower

*Foods for better brainpower*. (n.d.). Health.Harvard.

Retrieved 2018, from

https://www.health.harvard.edu/mind-and-

mood/foods-linked-to-better-brainpower

G.M. (2019b). *Benefits of strong triceps*. Healthline.

https://www.healthline.com/health/tricep-

kickbacks#:~:text=The%20triceps%20are%

20essential%20for,and%20increases%20ran

ge%20of%20motion

*Good vs Bad carbs.* (2017). Everydayhealth.

https://www.everydayhealth.com/diet-

nutrition/diet/good-carbs-bad-

carbs/#:~:text=The%20three%20main%20ty

pes%20of,for%20you%20and%20what's%2

0not

G.T. (2017c). *HIIT benefits.* Healthline.

https://www.healthline.com/nutrition/benefit

s-of-hiit#TOC_TITLE_HDR_3

*How to train HIIT.* (2018). Inbodyusa.

https://inbodyusa.com/blogs/inbodyblog/ho

w-to-use-hiit-to-improve-your-body-

composition/

J.C. (2019c). *Benefits of strong calves*.

Sportandspinalphysio.

https://sportandspinalphysio.com.au/the-

importance-of-calf-strength-and-the-best-

calf-strength-exercises/

*Mental benefits of exercise*. (n.d.). Waldenu.

https://www.waldenu.edu/online-bachelors-

programs/bs-in-psychology/resource/five-

mental-benefits-of-exercise

N. (2018d). *Why is a strong back important*.

Integrativeosteopathy.

https://integrativeosteopathy.com.au/build-strong-back-important/

N.B. (2020). *Essential nutrients*. Healthline. https://www.healthline.com/health/food-nutrition/six-essential-nutrients#vitamins

P.R. (2011). *The damage of alcohol*. Bbc. https://www.bbc.com/news/health-15114325#:~:text=Long%20term%2C%20it%20increases%20the,memory%20skills%20and%20reduce%20fertility

*Recovery tips*. (2018). Clevelandclinic. https://health.clevelandclinic.org/strenuous-workouts-try-these-6-best-recovery-tips/

R.L. (2018e). *Fat burning tips*. Healthline.

> https://www.healthline.com/nutrition/best-
> ways-to-burn-fat

S.H.Y. (n.d.-b). *Making more time in the day*.
Lifehack.

> https://www.lifehack.org/articles/featured/21
> -ways-to-add-more-hours-to-the-day.html

S.J. (2016). *Discomfort brings success*. Forbes.

> https://www.forbes.com/sites/sujanpatel/201
> 6/03/09/why-feeling-uncomfortable-is-the-
> key-to-success/?sh=5debcaa91913

*Using energy*. (n.d.). Memorialhermann.

> https://memorialhermann.org/services/specia
> lties/ironman-sports-medicine-